Child and Adolescent Anxiety Psychodynamic
Psychotherapy

Child and Adolescent Anxiety Psychodynamic Psychotherapy

A Treatment Manual

Sabina E. Preter, MD, PhD

Weill Cornell Medical College

New York, NY

Theodore Shapiro, MD

Weill Cornell Medical College

New York Presbyterian Hospital

New York, NY

Barbara Milrod, MD

Weill Cornell Medical College

New York Presbyterian Hospital

New York, NY

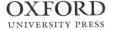

OXFORD

UNIVERSITY PRESS

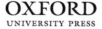

OXFORD
UNIVERSITY PRESS

Oxford University Press is a department of the University of Oxford. It furthers
the University's objective of excellence in research, scholarship, and education
by publishing worldwide. Oxford is a registered trade mark of Oxford University
Press in the UK and certain other countries.

Published in the United States of America by Oxford University Press
198 Madison Avenue, New York, NY 10016, United States of America.

© Oxford University Press 2018

CIP data is on file at the Library of Congress
ISBN 978–0–19–087771–2

1 3 5 7 9 8 6 4 2

Printed by WebCom, Inc., Canada

Give me a child until he is seven and I will show you the man—Aristotle

Contents

1

Introduction

Anxiety is universal and ubiquitous, but only about 30% of people, including children, are burdened with an anxiety disorder (1). Crippling anxiety in childhood and adolescence, if left unchecked, grows and casts a dark shadow on later development. This book will operationalize a relatively brief, accessible psychotherapy intervention for children and teens with anxiety disorders. It is a time-limited adaptation of a commonly practiced form of non–exposure-based, affect-focused, psychodynamic psychotherapy (2). The hope is to broaden the therapeutic armamentarium of operationalized psychotherapies for children and teens in order to minimize the burden of anxiety in childhood.

1.1. Rationale for CAPP

Child and adolescent anxiety psychodynamic psychotherapy (CAPP) is a time-limited, manualized psychodynamic psychotherapy treatment for children and adolescents aged 8 to 16 years suffering from a variety of anxiety disorders, including generalized anxiety disorder, separation anxiety disorder, social anxiety disorder, panic disorder, and comorbid posttraumatic stress disorder (PTSD). We have found this treatment to be useful in a small case series (3, 4), as well as relatively easy to implement by mental health clinicians with some amount of knowledge of psychodynamic principles and treatment who have been trained in this method. CAPP is a manualized psychotherapy that is individualized for each patient, yet it follows principles that are presented in this manual and is relatively easily taught and applied.

In this introductory chapter, we review the significance and impact of anxiety disorders in childhood. We then briefly review the current interventions used and describe the rationale for CAPP, elucidate its origins, give a synopsis of the main principles of treatment, and delineate its structure.

Children and teens with anxiety disorders are a large and clinically important population, and anxiety disorders are the most prevalent mental health disorders in youth. The combined prevalence of generalized anxiety disorder, separation anxiety disorder, and social phobia in youth is 15.4% (5, 6). Childhood anxiety disorders can be debilitating if untreated or partially treated. Youths risk continuing symptoms into adulthood and the development of major depression (1) and substance abuse disorders (7). Youngsters with anxiety disorders have an increased likelihood of suffering from more than one mental health condition. Suicide attempt rates are remarkably high: 14.3% for social phobia and 16.4% for generalized anxiety disorder across age (8).

In addition to the suffering of the child or teen, anxiety disorders have noticeable consequences for the family. A recent study of preschoolers with separation anxiety, generalized anxiety, and social phobia (9) describes how anxiety disorders in very young children affect families as well. The authors found that parents of children with early-onset anxiety disorders were 3.5 times more likely than parents of children who had developmentally expectable anxiety to report a negative impact on the four areas of finances, the ability to engage in activities, quality of relationships, and parents' well-being and mental health.

Kossowsky et al. (10) conducted a meta-analysis of 25 studies including 14,855 separation anxious children and found a convincing association between childhood separation anxiety disorder and later development of adult anxiety disorders, in particular panic disorder, but the results did not show an increased risk for depression and substance abuse. However, the latter sample size was small. Copeland et al. (11) suggest that generalized anxiety disorder alone accounts for the association between anxiety disorders and later depression (12).

The large population-based prospective study, the Great Smoky Mountains Study, by Copeland et al. (13) examined 1,420 children prospectively. The authors found high rates of separation anxiety disorder in younger children, less anxiety in older school-aged children, and an upsurge of social phobia, panic disorder, and agoraphobia in teenagers (14, 15). The transition from adolescence to young adulthood puts individuals at greatest risk for a diagnosis of an anxiety disorder. By their mid-20s more than one in five individuals carried a diagnosis of an anxiety disorder (1) (28.8% lifetime in the National Comorbidity Survey Replication [NCSR]). Each individual childhood anxiety disorder was associated with adverse functioning in at least one young adult functional domain, such as health outcome, financial outcome, and interpersonal functioning. Generalized anxiety disorder and *Diagnostic and Statistical Manual of Mental Disorders, third edition, revised* (DSM-III-R) overanxious disorder were associated with poor functioning in all domains, separation anxiety disorder was associated with poor health outcomes, and social anxiety disorder was associated with significant interpersonal problems.

Anxiety can be transmitted from one generation to the next (16). This transmission is thought to occur because of biological and genetic vulnerabilities as well as epigenetic (environmental) factors, parental behaviors, and often subtle verbal as well as nonverbal communications to the child. A central example is separation anxiety disorder. Separation-anxious children often have parents who themselves have been struggling with separation anxiety for many years. A common presentation is a school-aged child who refuses to sleep in his/her own bed, at a time and place in which family culture and the larger culture would expect the child to do so. Parents who present with now modified but nevertheless ongoing separation anxiety may feel unable to soothe the child's distress or to limit agitation unless they acquiesce to anxious demands, which aggravates the child's difficulty in relinquishing the symptom. They often feel particularly uncomfortable not acceding to the child's anxiously fueled wishes.

Undiagnosed and untreated anxiety disorders contribute to increased and perhaps unnecessary health care utilization, well known from studies in adults with anxiety disorders (NCSR: 42.3 billion annually) (17). In youth, this occurs in part as a result of somatic symptoms anxious children experience (18), in the absence of a diagnosed medical condition, or in excess of what would typically be expected in the course of a diagnosed medical illness. Cardiac symptoms (rapid heartbeat and chest pain), respiratory symptoms (shortness of breath), gastrointestinal symptoms (nausea, vomiting, abdominal pain, and diarrhea), and neurological symptoms (dizziness and headaches) are commonly reported, particularly among children whose anxiety disorders are not properly diagnosed and treated. The child or teen may undergo unnecessary diagnostic procedures as well as otherwise avoidable medical treatments. The cost offset of earlier proper identification and treatment is large.

A limited number of evidence-based treatments have been adequately tested for efficacy, namely cognitive-behavioral therapy (CBT) and antianxiety medications, primarily selective serotonin reuptake inhibitors (SSRIs). CBT treatment is thought to work by exposure to feared situations (exposure-response-prevention), except in adolescents, in whom stage-related brain development is thought to interfere (19, 20). Elements of typical CBT protocols include psychoeducation, cognitive restructuring, relaxation training, and exposure to feared stimuli, often repeated in homework that is monitored.

CBT and medication are effective treatments. In the Child/Adolescent Anxiety Multimodal Study (CAMS) (21, 22), 60% responded to CBT alone and 55% to SSRI alone. Nonetheless, more than 40% of anxious children and adolescents do not respond to medication or CBT alone. When combined, medication and CBT have higher response rates at treatment termination (80.7%, but decreases to 45.6 at follow-up) (23), but limiting factors of CBT arise when patients may be unwilling to expose themselves to feared situations and are reluctant to complete necessary homework assignments, both of which decrease treatment efficacy (24).

Medication use, primarily SSRIs, has increased in children with a positive risk-benefit ratio of SSRIs (25, 26). However, reports of increased suicidal ideation and behavior on SSRIs (27) have compounded some parents' and physicians' reluctance to allow children to take medication (28). Many patients with anxiety disorders prefer psychotherapy to medication, as parents of children with anxiety disorders often do.

It would be beneficial if the parents of pediatric anxiety patients had a choice of efficacious psychosocial interventions, which would allow acknowledging personal preferences for different treatment approaches and potentially different types of patients with different response profiles. Systematic study of alternative treatments can help identify which type of intervention works better for whom and will potentially clarify underlying mechanisms, which may in turn illuminate fundamentals of anxiety in childhood. Thus, although evidence-based treatments such as medications and CBT are available, there is ample justification to establish alternative interventions, which can then be assessed as to their evidentiary basis, to accommodate the needs of other families and children and allow access to a tailored match of treatment.

CAPP is distinguishable from CBT in that it fosters a deeper psychological understanding of the meaning of the child's anxiety symptoms. This process occurs verbally or in play by reworking anxious memories and associations, making them accessible to modification using techniques other than exposure/response-prevention that are focused on improving dysregulated attachment and promoting and ideally normalizing reflective functioning (29). CAPP relates anxiety symptoms to underlying emotional meanings of conflicts operating outside of children's awareness. This helps patients to access and better define their emotional understandings, focuses on better articulation and subsequent sense of mastery over dysregulated and excessive emotional activation in relation to attachments, and helps promote a sense of safety to act autonomously in the world. Such approaches appeal to a child's reflective function and personal sense of coherence.

The ability to think about one's own mind is referred to as "reflective function" (see Chapter 2, Section 2.2), a normative developmental capacity that can be fostered and developed during psychotherapy with subsequent better understanding of the meaning of one's own and others' thoughts, emotions, and actions. This allows individuals treated with this method to use the acquired insights in the future. For example, a socially inhibited child beset with anxiety who cannot speak up in class can be helped by reflecting on her tendency to believe that 100% accuracy in performance is required in order to be loved and respected.

An advantage of this manualized psychodynamic treatment approach is that it can relatively easily be taught to clinicians with moderate levels of psychodynamic psychotherapy knowledge.

1.2. Psychoanalysis, Dynamic Psychotherapy, and Symptom-Focused Psychotherapy: Background and Comparisons

It may be said that Freud invented psychoanalysis during the last decade of the 19th century and continued to revise its tenets into the early 1930s. What has happened since may be taken as derivative paths that grew out of the foundational experience of the original group of psychoanalysts (30). Freud himself made major changes in his theory and practice as he came upon obstacles or new clinical phenomena that required revision. Among these shifts were the recognition of transference as a tool rather than only being seen as a resistance to therapy, the introduction of aggression as a primary drive to match sexuality, the structural theory (id, ego, and super ego) was added to the topographic theory (conscious / unconscious), and others. In addition, practical changes occurred, such as the use of the couch and the turn away from hypnosis to free association, as well as the change from the brief time spent in psychoanalysis of the early cases to longer treatments that focused more on personality change than on symptom alleviation. These internal alterations would provide a basis for future changes that were not possible during Freud's time with its struggle to preserve the "psychoanalytic revolution."

More specific to this manual, during the 1920s and thereafter, the psychoanalytic model was applied to children and adolescents, requiring further alterations of what had seemed a specific method by which the psychoanalyst plumbed the unconscious and sought discovery of the meanings of symptoms and the salience of defenses. Among the many developmental modifications of technique was a substitution of play for free association as an open-ended approach to uncovering underlying emotional content and meaning (31, 32, 33). The number of sessions per week and the observational stance that the therapist took remained similar. Practitioners who followed Anna Freud held regular visits with parents who reported the context of daily life to the psychoanalyst, who could use such information in tandem with the child's play. These sources of information served as a basis for interpretations of meaning to help the child improve coping. Thus the beginnings of child psychoanalysis represented a breach from psychoanalytic practice with adult patients in the service of exploring meanings derived from the child's psyche as connected with his/her real life as reported by another person. The technique was adapted to the task.

Psychodynamic psychotherapy and manualized psychotherapies, among other modifications, originated during the latter half of the 20th century. One could argue that some of Freud's early analyses were psychodynamic psychotherapies or psychodynamic consultations, such as his Katharina case (34).

Some of the older generation of psychoanalysts have broken ranks completely and supplanted psychodynamic therapies with their own brand names and practices. Beck (35) stands out as the original proponent of a new therapy, CBT, originally also an open-ended psychotherapeutic treatment, which has had a significant role in launching evidence-based treatments, as is the case for interpersonal psychotherapy (IPT) (36, 37). Researchers such as Mufson (38, 39) have adapted IPT for adolescents.

The subsequent advent of randomized controlled trials that were the gold standard of pharmacological studies seriously challenged the use of psychotherapy treatments and called for studies of efficacy. CBT is relatively easier to operationalize and dismantle by components than affect-focused psychotherapies and offers more generalized rules (true do's and don'ts) and sequences of interventions that convert much of the psychotherapy experience to learning strategies. It is necessary to examine how the current manualized psychodynamic and symptom-focused psychodynamic treatments still represent a variant of the original psychoanalysis and **continue to feature the aim of understanding the unconscious psychological meanings of symptoms and explication of narrative themes confounded by defensive avoidance. These aims require a self reflective grasp of one's own unconscious operations and fantasies**.

Freud's earliest case descriptions were brief treatments, focused on symptoms. Davanloo (40), Mann (41), and others during the 1970s and later also had clear psychodynamic aims, such as separation anxiety, conceived as a core issue in the treatment approach. These brief psychodynamic treatments required fewer sessions than the psychoanalytic prescription of four or five visits per week. These time-limited, but not manualized, dynamic therapies were never well adapted in a systematic way to children. However, many child psychiatrists did apply dynamic psychotherapies that were not psychoanalysis, employing play during one or two visits per week (42). The Anna Freud Center in London pioneered the experiment of fewer visits per week for children. These treatments depended on parental participation and were briefer and more focused. They were not subject to the rigor of manualization and differentiation from other psychotherapies, nor were they subjected to clinical trials of efficacy. These interventions were the most used approaches in children with "neurotic" symptoms during the second half of the 20th century, including those with anxiety disorders. Target and Fonagy (42) studied the Anna Freud Center cases retrospectively ($n = 763$) and sorted the differential outcomes in relation to diagnoses (disruptive disorders and anxiety/depressive disorders, either alone or combined), session frequency, and duration of treatment and developmental stage of the patient. The patients who improved most were those with anxiety disorders.

The notion of manualized, time-limited psychotherapies applied to specific disorders arrived later for children than adults. This manual is a relatively new and rare event in the psychotherapy arena for children, in that very few psychodynamic treatments for children have been operationalized. Kernberg and Chazan (43), and recently Hoffman, Rice, and Prout (44), offered publications of psychodynamic psychotherapies directed to youth with conduct disorders and behavioral impulse control disorders. However, neither group has published pilot outcome studies to date.

It is important to examine how this time-limited psychodynamic psychotherapy is related to the principles of child psychoanalysis. The frame is different because the treatment maintains *temporal limits and is conducted at a lower, twice-weekly, frequency. Parents are included,* but on an as-needed basis. The treatment is directed toward the meaning of symptoms, obeys the structural inquiry into defense mechanisms and transferences, and probes for significant unconscious constellations that drive symptoms and problematic behavior. These latter practices are derived from psychodynamic theory.

This manualized description provides an operationalized approach to children's behavior and psyche that draws on this rich recent movement while maintaining a core focus on the analysis of meaning.

1.3. CAPP: A Developmentally Modified Version of Panic-Focused Psychodynamic Psychotherapy

CAPP has been developed for children and adolescents with anxiety disorders and is a developmentally adapted version of panic-focused psychodynamic psychotherapy (PFPP) (45, 46), the only psychodynamic psychotherapy for panic disorder with demonstrated efficacy in adults.

PFPP combines psychoanalytic principles with a time-limited, symptom-focused treatment approach. It is the most rigorously studied form of dynamic therapy for anxiety disorders in adults (2, 45, 46, 47, 48). PFPP was tested in four (three published, one in process) randomized controlled trials and was found efficacious for panic disorder with or without agoraphobia in adults. PFPP has been readily adopted by dynamically oriented clinicians (47, 48), and its potential application beyond research settings has been demonstrated by successful dissemination to at least 12 clinical groups/clinics in the United States and Europe.

PFPP's clinical utility and adaptation to a range of anxiety disorders (49) suggested that a developmentally modified form might be a promising treatment approach for anxious youth.

While PFPP was initially conceptualized specifically for panic disorder, CAPP was specifically adapted to treat generalized anxiety disorder, separation anxiety disorder, and social anxiety disorder, conditions that share disabling anxious preoccupations and features of anticipatory anxiety and avoidance, although they differ in specific fear foci and corresponding situational avoidance. These disorders were chosen in order to develop a psychodynamic intervention that could be tested and compared with the most commonly utilized CBT intervention for youth anxiety disorders, Coping Cat (50).

The central therapeutic elements and techniques of PFPP that were tailored to a younger patient population are its *focus on personal meanings of anxiety symptoms*. They are gleaned from organized, yet relatively unstructured, gathering of data from the patient's narratives. Regardless of age, this dynamic therapy postulates that anxiety symptoms and avoidance carry specific psychological meanings that are at least in part unconscious, unique to each patient. For symptoms to exert a significant emotional pull, their significance exists at least in part outside of the patient's awareness.

Examples of areas that require age-related adaptation in CAPP compared with PFPP are involvement of parents/caretakers, consideration of the developmental stage of the child/teen with subsequent adaptation to his/her emotional, cognitive, and linguistic maturity, and consideration of various vehicles of communication in session, such as play, drawing, and talk.

Thus far CAPP has been tested in a small open, pilot clinical trial (3, 4). CAPP is a 24-session, 12-week, manualized psychodynamic psychotherapy. The open trial was conducted in 10 patients aged eight to 16 years with primary generalized anxiety disorder, social phobia, and/or separation anxiety disorder. Patients with comorbid depression, obsessive compulsive disorder (OCD), attention deficit hyperactivity disorder (ADHD), and other anxiety disorders, such as panic disorder and comorbid PTSD, were included. Patients with psychosis; bipolar disorder; acute suicidality; current substance dependence; organic mental syndromes; acute, severe, unstable medical conditions; autistic spectrum disorders; and mental retardation were excluded. All study subjects were fluent in English. No patient was on anti-anxiety medication.

Study benchmarks, including inclusion/exclusion criteria, outcome measures, and definitions of response, were designed to match those of the CAMS (22). The goal was to determine whether psychodynamic psychotherapy has a clinical impact on subjects who met CAMS criteria. The results showed that of the nine subjects who completed the treatment (there was one dropout), all improved across all measured outcome domains at treatment termination, and results were sustained at six months' follow-up, without intervening treatment.

These are encouraging results, which suggest that CAPP merits further testing in a randomized controlled trial in order to determine whether this treatment can play a role as an alternative treatment for youth anxiety disorders.

1.4. Cases: Fourteen-Year-Old Marie and Thirteen-Year-Old Tom

We offer introductions to two CAPP psychotherapies that were conducted in accord with the CAPP manual. We present the narratives of early, middle, and final phases of the treatments of 14-year-old Marie and 13-year-old Tom so that readers may follow the course and interventions in clinical examples that apply the treatment described in this manual.

1.4.1. Marie's Initial Presentation

Marie was a 14-year-old ninth-grader who presented with a two-and-a-half-year history of severe anxiety, including episodes of dizziness, crying, and inability to speak in situations outside of her home or school classes. She was essentially homebound, other than attending school, for fear of having to interact with peers or "even adults," including the neighbors she had known for years. The idea of running an errand at a convenience store near her home felt unreachable. She hid the severity of her crippling anxiety with her parents. She felt desperate, trapped, and incompetent and resorted to cutting her wrists and legs to relieve tension, accompanied by thoughts of dying by suicide.

Marie came from a close-knit, religious family and was shy growing up. At school, she was teased for being (culturally) "different," as well as for looking different from her peers at school. During middle school, particularly seventh and eighth grades, the "teasing" from peers escalated to vicious bullying by almost the whole class on most school days. She was physically assaulted by a former elementary school friend, who had turned against her and had become the ringleader of her assailants. Marie never fought back and denied the assault to her parents, even though it was witnessed by a neighbor. She only mentioned casually to her mother that she wanted to switch schools, not saying how much she was suffering, and her mother did not realize what the real reason for her saying this was. Marie continued to suffer, sobbing herself to sleep most nights. She was greatly relieved when she changed to a high school of her choice, away from the bullies, and she had the fantasy that she would leave all her problems behind because she had left her tormentors. To her surprise, however, her anxiety grew worse in the new school. Her inability to venture into public spaces increased further, and she had intrusive thoughts of being ridiculed if she needed to speak at all. One day Marie refused to go into a bookstore while her mother waited in the car, but her mother tried to force her. Marie collapsed into tears, admitting to her mother how terrified she was to go anywhere or speak to anyone, even if it was only to speak to a salesperson to help her find the book she needed. At this point, her mother finally learned about the severity of Marie's social phobia and agoraphobia and brought her for treatment.

Marie's DSM-IV diagnoses at evaluation on the Anxiety Disorders Interview Schedule, Child and Parent Version (51) were: social phobia 7/8, agoraphobia 6/8, separation anxiety disorder 4/8, and PTSD from severe bullying in middle school 4/8.

1.4.2. Tom's Initial Presentation

Tom was a 13-year-old seventh-grader who had been diagnosed with a mild nonverbal learning disability, dysthymic disorder, social phobia, and separation anxiety. He had a long-standing history of shyness, inhibitions, and phobias. When Tom started treatment in the CAPP study, his most salient symptoms were constant worries about his school performance, his peer relations, food allergies, bodily complaints, concerns about attracting illnesses, and about "getting things right." He had a fear of the dark and persistent separation anxiety with worries about his family's well-being, and he avoided new experiences because he was worried about what peers might think of him. His nonverbal learning disability was mild, but his constant anxiety about his school performance heightened his learning difficulties. He was well liked by his teachers, and his parents described him as pliable and "too good." This contrasted with his subjective experience of life being so stressful that he often felt, "I hate my life and wish I was someone else." Three months before starting treatment Tom was robbed by an older youth who stole his wallet.

From a very early age, Tom was "slow to warm up," shy, a "worrier." He had separation anxiety when he started preschool. His mother also described that it was hard for her to let him go. He did not talk spontaneously in school, and his pretend play was limited. This resulted in his participation in small-group play therapy at the age of four with some improvement. In kindergarten and elementary school, he continued to be very shy, did not participate, and was very slow to develop friendships. It was not until middle school that Tom began to engage more with peers.

Before starting CAPP, Tom worked briefly with a CBT therapist but did not find it helpful.

Tom's DSM-IV diagnoses at evaluation on the Anxiety Disorders Interview Schedule, Child and Parent Version (51) were: social phobia 6/8, separation anxiety disorder 5/8, and dysthymic disorder 4/8.

We will follow Marie and Tom throughout this volume to demonstrate the ways in which their respective CAPP treatments unfolded.

1.5. Overview of the Three Phases of Treatment

Conceptually, CAPP is divided into three phases: opening phase, middle phase, and termination phase, each about eight sessions long. Practically, in the office, these phases transition seamlessly into one another and often overlap. Throughout the treatment, the technique resembles an open-ended psychodynamic psychotherapy approach because the patient is free to pursue his/her thoughts in an unstructured manner during sessions, but the therapist keeps the presenting anxiety symptoms in mind at all times and gently but consistently redirects the patient to focus on the underlying emotional meanings of his/her anxiety.

The central psychoanalytic principle that there is meaning and significance that determine anxiety symptoms, with the therapist as guide to its understanding, supports the claim that this is a symptom-focused psychodynamic psychotherapy.

1.5.1. Opening Phase—Treatment of Acute Anxiety

After taking the patient's history of anxiety symptoms and associated events with the parents of younger children alone and, if desired, with the parents *and* adolescent-aged patient present, the patient/therapist dyad begins to meet alone. The aim of the first few sessions is to achieve empathic and attentive cooperative rapport between patient and therapist and to begin to identify specific psychological dynamisms as underlying the child's anxiety symptoms that need to be understood. Based on the psychoanalytic premise that the meaning of anxiety symptoms can be understood as a window into otherwise inaccessible aspects of mental life, the therapist helps the patient to explore circumstances and feelings surrounding anxiety onset, personal psychological meanings of specific anxiety symptoms, and feelings and content of anxiety episodes.

As the therapist listens to the play or talk narrative the child develops, core conflicts around the following themes typically emerge:

1. *Separation and autonomy* with *ambivalence* about becoming age-appropriately independent. This can be a conflict within the individual child's own mind, but also can be a conflict within the family, with the parent having difficulties letting the child begin to separate. This is a common dynamism in separation anxiety disorder, panic disorder, and agoraphobia/avoidance. Difficulties separating often relate to *ambivalent relationships* with close attachment figures. Much attention is paid during sessions

to the emotional impact of both early and ongoing relationships and their conflicts, including difficulties tolerating anger at close attachment figures. Relationships with important attachment figures are central, and the core emotional aspects of these relationships are often repeated in the context of the therapeutic relationship and expressed in the transference (see Glossary).

2. Difficulties experiencing and expressing *anger or rage* and *mixed loving and aggressive* feelings is another common psychological dynamism, often seen in panic disorder and generalized anxiety disorder, PTSD and agoraphobia, wherein the individual has to be hypervigilant all the time out of an unconscious fear of losing control of his/her own aggressive or sexual urges.

3. Highly charged, *conflicted feelings over desire for admiration and display*, as well as *conflicted sexual fantasies*, can lead to social removal and social phobia, as well as guilty self-punishment, which can be enacted through anxiety symptoms and their consequences.

It is essential that at least one core dynamic conflict underlying the anxiety symptoms be verbally identified to the patient early in therapy, no later than session 4 or 5. These conflicts must be articulated very specifically because they refer to experience-near events and feelings as the child expresses them. This dynamism is often just one of a few that operate together, and *CAPP is "dynamic" both in terms of its form and in terms of the dynamic elaboration and further modification of its formulation in response to additional information that is uncovered about meanings of anxiety as treatment unfolds.*

To summarize, the opening phase of CAPP serves to establish rapport with the family and the child/teen, followed by a largely unstructured technique, with particular attention to and focus on the very specific details of the presenting anxiety symptoms. The main task for this phase is to collaboratively identify the psychological dynamisms underlying the patient's symptoms, although this initial formulation is often amended as treatment progresses.

1.5.2. Middle Phase—Working Through and Treatment of Anxiety Vulnerability

The central dynamisms that are identified in the opening phase are addressed repeatedly as they are recognized as recurrent themes in the dialogue and are worked through, exploring the ways these conflicts affect various aspects of the patient's life. The therapist maintains his/her open-ended attitude but focuses on the symptoms and associated core conflicts, tracking symptoms in real time alongside intercurrent emotional events in the child's life. This emphasizes the patient as a participant and collaborator with the therapist in the task of uncovering the meanings of maladaptive anxious phenomena.

During the middle phase of treatment, these central dynamisms are revisited focally and recognized in their many representations during the therapy. These manifestations are the surface phenomenology that warrant and yield to improvement in reflective functioning as the child is made aware of how he/she has been self-protecting, for example, from experiencing shame and/or guilt as core fantasies are exposed, articulated and better understood.

Main techniques are determining emotional meanings and language surrounding the anxiety experience and consistently addressing defense mechanisms, which function to protect the individual from overwhelming anxiety but are ultimately maladaptive. The same set of emotional conflicts typically emerge across many settings; one of these settings is often the relationship with the therapist, which allows a therapeutic "working through" in real time. In this way, core relationship patterns and feeling constructs can be understood verbally and discussed, rather than yet again having the child burdened by a simple re-enactment of the same pattern.

This identification and exploration of emotionally conflicted affects, ideas, and fantasies that trigger anxiety symptoms help the child/teen to grasp the heretofore immaturely fixed meanings of these anxiety symptoms. As a result, the anxiety symptoms become more plastic and amenable to change.

The therapist aids the patient in articulating thoughts and feelings related to the transference and helps the child to begin to understand its meaning. We hypothesize that this specifically aids in the improvement of reflective functioning, which has been postulated to be a common feature of dynamic treatment efficacy (29, 52, 53, 54).

Ultimately, articulating and understanding the meanings and emotional underpinnings of these core conflicts and anxiety symptoms allows for acknowledgement, familiarity, and symptomatic change.

1.5.3. Termination Phase

During the final phase, the therapeutic work continues and the focus on dynamisms underlying anxiety remains, while preparing the child to resume his/her life tasks at home, in school, and with peers after therapy has ended. The expectation is to be freed of the burden of symptoms that inhibit and constrain action and enable the child to enter life's arena with a greater degree of adaptive freedom. *The therapist must bring up termination of therapy and actively address how the child feels about it, whether the child brings it up or not, for the final third (8 sessions) of the treatment.*

Core separation/autonomy and ambivalent rage conflicts are often re-experienced as the treatment comes to an end. This permits children and adolescents to again recognize and articulate these feelings directly in the relationship to the therapist. This phase of treatment is very important. A temporary recurrence of symptoms as these feelings are experienced with the therapist during termination can occur. The patient now demonstrates his/her new ability to manage separations, relationships, and independence, this time in a verbal, rather than in a symptomatic, form.

The therapeutic work enhances the child's ability to reflect, and symptomatic anxiety can be warded off by mental grasp of the emotional meanings of the symptoms. The treatment aims are to broaden horizons and the child's scope of possible thought and behavior and to allow less inhibited action and better anxiety tolerance as well as a better grasp of the meaning of symptoms.

Just as Bowlby (55) suggested that attachment serves the toddler's aim to explore the world from a safe internal base, the therapy seeks to serve a similar purpose so that anxiety is no longer crippling but instead becomes a signal of danger rather than a nidus of symptom formation or a reason for inhibition.

References

1. Kessler, R. C., Berglund, P., Demler, O., Jin, R., Merikangas, K. R., & Walters, E. E. (2005). Lifetime prevalence and age-of-onset distributions of DSM-IV disorders in the National Comorbidity Survey Replication. *Archives of General Psychiatry, 62*(6), 593–602.

2. Busch, F. N., Milrod, B. L., Singer, M. B., & Aronson, A. C. (2011). *Manual of panic focused psychodynamic psychotherapy—eXtended range.* New York, NY: Routledge.

3. Milrod, B., Shapiro, T., Gross, C., Silver, G., Preter, S., Libow, A., & Leon, A. C. (2013). Does manualized psychodynamic psychotherapy have an impact on youth anxiety disorders? *American Journal of Psychotherapy, 67*(4), 359–366.

4. Silver, G., Shapiro, T., & Milrod, B. (2013). Treatment of anxiety in children and adolescents using child and adolescent anxiety psychodynamic psychotherapy. *Child and Adolescent Psychiatric Clinics of North America, 22*(1), 83–96.

5. Kessler, R. C., Chiu, W. T., Demler, O., Merikangas, K. R., & Walters, E. E. (2005). Prevalence, severity, and comorbidity of 12-month DSM-IV disorders in the National Comorbidity Survey Replication. *Archives of General Psychiatry, 62*(6), 617–627.

6. Shear, K., Jin, R., Ruscio, A. M., Walters, E. E., & Kessler, R. C. (2006). Prevalence and correlates of estimated DSM-IV child and adult separation anxiety disorder in the National Comorbidity Survey Replication. *American Journal of Psychiatry, 163*(6), 1074–1083.

7. Regier, D. A., Rae, D. S., Narrow, W. E., Kaelber, C. T., & Schatzberg, A. F. (1998). Prevalence of anxiety disorders and their comorbidity with mood and addictive disorders. *British Journal of Psychiatry Supplement, 34,* 24–28.

8. Milrod, B., Busch, F., Cooper, A., & Shapiro, T. (1997). *Manual of panic-focused psychodynamic psychotherapy.* Washington, DC: American Psychiatric Association Press.

9. Towe-Goodman, N. R., Franz, L., Copeland, W., Angold, A., & Egger, H. (2014). Perceived family impact of preschool anxiety disorders. *Journal of the American Academy of Child and Adolescent Psychiatry, 53*(4), 437–446.

10. Kossowsky, J., Pfaltz, M. C., Schneider, S., Taeymans, J., Locher, C., & Gaab, J. (2013). The separation anxiety hypothesis of panic disorder revisited: A meta-analysis. *American Journal of Psychiatry, 170*(7), 768–781.

11. Copeland, W. E., Shanahan, L., Costello, E. J., & Angold, A. (2009). Childhood and adolescent psychiatric disorders as predictors of young adult disorders. *Archives of General Psychiatry, 66*(7), 764–772.

12. Britton, J. C., Lissek, S., Grillon, C., Norcross, M. A., & Pine, D. S. (2011). Development of anxiety: The role of threat appraisal and fear learning. *Depression and Anxiety, 28*(1), 5–17.

13. Copeland, W. E., Angold, A., Shanahan, K., & Costello, E. J. (2014). Longitudinal patterns of anxiety from childhood to adulthood: The Great Smoky Mountains Study. *Journal of the American Academy of Child and Adolescent Psychiatry, 53*(1), 21–33.

14. Biederman, J., Faraone, S. V., Marrs, A., Moore, P., Garcia, J., Ablon, S., . . . Kearns, M. E. (1997). Panic disorder and agoraphobia in consecutively referred children and adolescents. *Journal of the American Academy of Child and Adolescent Psychiatry, 36*(2), 214–223.

15. Hansen, C., Sanders, S. L., Massaro, S., & Last, C. G. (1998). Predictors of severity of absenteeism in children with anxiety-based school refusal. *Journal of Clinical Child Psychology, 27*(3), 246–254.

16. Milrod, B., Markowitz, J. C., Gerber, A., Cyranowski, J., Altemus, M., Shapiro, T., . . . Glatt, C. (2014). Childhood separation anxiety and the pathogenesis and treatment of adult anxiety. *American Journal of Psychiatry, 171,* 34–43.

17. Greenberg, P. E., Sisistky, T., Kessler, R. C., Finkelstein, S. N., Berndt, E. R., Davidson, J. R., . . . Fyer, A. J. (1999). The economic burden of anxiety disorders in the 1990s. *Journal of Clinical Psychiatry, 60*(7), 427–435.

18. Ramsawh, H. J., Chavira, D. A., & Stein, M. B. (2010). Burden of anxiety disorders in pediatric medical settings: Prevalence, phenomenology, and a research agenda. *Archives of Pediatrics and Adolescent Medicine, 164*(10), 965–972.

19. Patwell, S. S., Duhoux, S., & Hartley, C. A. (2012). Altered fear learning across development in both mouse and human. *Proceedings of the National Academy of Science USA, 109*(40), 16318–16323.

20. Johnson, D. C., & Casey, B. J. (2015). Easy to remember, difficult to forget. *Developmental Cognitive Neuroscience, 11*, 42–55.

21. Walkup, J. T., Albano, A. M., Piacentini, J., Birmaher, B., Compton, S. N., Sherrill, J. T., . . . Kendall, P. C. (2008). Cognitive behavioral therapy, sertraline, or a combination in childhood anxiety. *New England Journal of Medicine, 359*(26), 2753–2766.

22. Compton, S. N, Walkup, J. T., Albano, A. M., Piacentini, A. C., Birmaher, B., Sherrill, J. T., . . . March, J. S. (2010). Child/Adolescent Anxiety Multimodal Study (CAMS): Rationale, design, and methods. *Child and Adolescent Psychiatry and Mental Health, 4*, 1.

23. Ginsburg, G. S., Becker, E. M., Keeton, C. P., Sakolsky, D., Piacentini, J., Albano, A. M., . . . Kendall, P. C. (2014). Naturalistic follow-up of youths treated for pediatric anxiety disorders. *Journal of the American Medical Association Psychiatry, 71*(3), 310–318.

24. Fernandez, E., Salem, D., Swift, J. K., & Ramtahal, N. (2015). Meta-analysis of dropout from cognitive behavioral therapy: Magnitude, timing, and moderators. *Journal of Consulting and Clinical Psychology, 83*(6), 1108–1122.

25. Birmaher, B., Axelson, D. A., Monk, K., Kalas, C., Clark, D. B., Ehmann, M., . . . Brent, D. A. (2003). Fluoxetine for the treatment of childhood anxiety disorders. *Journal of the American Academy of Child and Adolescent Psychiatry, 42*(4), 415–423.

26. Rynn, M. A., Siqueland, L., & Rickels, K. (2008). Placebo-controlled trial of sertraline in the treatment of children with generalized anxiety disorders. *American Journal of Psychiatry, 158*(12), 2008–2014.

27. *FDA statement on recommendations of the Psychopharmacologic Drugs and Pediatric Advisory Committees.* (2004, September 16). Retrieved from http://childadvocate.net/fda-and-antidepressants-in-children/.

28. Lu, C. Y., Zhang, F., Lakoma, M. D., Madden, J. M., Rusinak, D., Penfold, R. B., . . . Soumerai, S. B. (2014). Changes in antidepressant use by young people and suicidal behavior after FDA warnings and media coverage: Quasi-experimental study. *British Medical Journal, 348*, g3596.

29. Fonagy, P., & Bateman, A. (2008). The development of borderline personality disorder: A mentalizing model. *Journal of Personality Disorders, 22*, 4–21.

30. Makari, G. (2008). *Revolution in mind.* New York, NY: Harper Perennial.

31. Hug-Hellmuth, H. V. (1921). On the technique of child analysis. *International Journal of Psychoanalysis, 2*, 287–296.

32. Klein, M. (1932). *The psychoanalysis of children* (*International Psycho-Analytic Library*, Vol. 22, pp. 1–379). London, UK: The Hogarth Press.

33. Freud, A. (1954). Psychoanalysis and education. *Psychoanalytic Study of the Child 9;9*–15.

34. Freud, S. (1893). *Katharina, case histories from studies on hysteria* (Standard ed., Vol. 2, pp. 125–134). London, UK: The Hogarth Press.

35. Beck, A. (1975). *Cognitive therapy and the emotional disorders.* Madison, CT: International Universities Press.

36. Klerman, G. L., Weissman, M. M., Rounsaville, B. J., & Chevron, E. S. (1984). *Interpersonal psychotherapy of depression.* New York, NY: Basic Books.

37. Weissman, M. M., Markowitz, J. W., & Klerman, G. L. (2000). *The guide to interpersonal psychotherapy* (updated and expanded ed.). New York, NY: Oxford University Press.

38. Mufson, L. H., Pollack Dorta, K., Moreau, D., & Weissman, M. M. (2011). *Interpersonal psychotherapy for depressed adolescents* (2nd ed.). New York, NY: Guilford Press.

39. Young, J. F., Makover, H. B., Cohen, J. R., Mufson, L., Gallop, R. J., & Benas, J. S. (2012). Interpersonal psychotherapy-adolescent skills training: Anxiety outcomes and impact of comorbidity. *Journal of Clinical Child and Adolescent Psychology, 41*(5), 640–653.

40. Davanloo, H. (1977). *Short-term dynamic psychotherapy.* Lanham, MD: Jason Aronson.

41. Mann, J. (1980). *Time-limited psychotherapy.* Cambridge, MA: Harvard University Press.

42. Target, M., & Fonagy, P. (1994). Efficacy of psychoanalysis for children with emotional disorders. *Journal of the American Academy of Child and Adolescent Psychiatry, 33*(3), 361–371.

43. Kernberg, P. F., & Chazan, S. E. (1991). *Children with conduct disorders: A psychotherapy manual.* New York, NY: Basic Books.

44. Hoffman, L., Rice, T., & Prout, T. (2015). *Manual of regulation-focused psychotherapy for children (RFP-C) with externalizing behaviors.* London, UK: Routledge.

45. Milrod, B., Busch, F., Cooper, A., & Shapiro, T. (1997). *Manual of panic-focused psychodynamic psychotherapy.* Washington, DC: American Psychiatric Association Press.

46. Milrod, B., Leon, A. C., Busch, F., Rudden, M., Schwalberg, M., Clarkin, J., . . . Shear, M. K. (2007). A randomized controlled clinical trial of psychoanalytic psychotherapy for panic disorder. *American Journal of Psychiatry, 164,* 265–272.

47. Beutel, M., Scheurich, V., Knebel, A., Michal, M., Wiltink, J., Graf-Morgenstern, M., . . . Subic-Wrana, C. (2013). Implementing panic-focused psychodynamic psychotherapy into clinical practice. *Canadian Journal of Psychiatry, 58*(6), 326–334.

48. Sandell, R., Svensson, M., Nilsson, T., Johansson, H., Viborg, G., & Perrin, S. (2015). The POSE study—panic control treatment versus panic-focused psychodynamic psychotherapy under randomized and self-selection conditions: Study protocol for a randomized controlled trial. *Trials, 16,* 130.

49. Milrod, B., Altemus, M., Gross, C., Busch, F., Silver, G., Christos, P., . . . Schneier, F. (2016). Adult separation anxiety in treatment nonresponders with anxiety disorders: Delineation of the syndrome and exploration of attachment-based psychotherapy and biomarkers. *Comprehensive Psychiatry, 66,* 139–145.

50. Kendall, P. C., & Hedtke, K. A. (2006). *Coping cat workbook* (2nd ed.). Ardmore, PA: Workbook Publishing.

51. Silverman, W. K., & Albano, A. M. (2004). *Anxiety Disorders Interview Schedule (ADIS-IV): Child and Parent Version.* New York, NY: Oxford University Press and Graywind Publications.

52. Ekeblad, A., Falkenstroem, F., & Holmqvist, R. (2016). Reflective functioning as predictor of working alliance and outcome in the treatment of depression. *Journal of Consulting and Clinical Psychology, 84*(1), 67–78.

53. Milrod, B., Chambless, D. L., Gallop, R., Busch, F. N., Schwalberg, M., McCarthy, K. S., . . . Barber, J. P. (2016). Psychotherapies for panic disorder: A tale of two sites. *Journal of Clinical Psychiatry, 77*(7), 927–935.

54. Rudden, M. G., Milrod, B., Meehan, K. M., & Falkenstrom, F. (2009). Symptom-specific reflective functioning: Incorporating psychoanalytic measures into clinical trials. *Journal of the American Psychoanalytic Association, 57*(6), 1473–1478.

55. Bowlby, J. (1958). The nature of the child's tie to his mother. *International Journal of Psychoanalysis, 39,* 350–373.

2

Time-Limited Psychodynamic Psychotherapy

2.1. Theory and Clinical Issues

The idea of a manualized dynamic psychotherapy for children and adolescents was not always easy to imagine because children are less behaviorally predictable than adults and psychodynamic therapy is often practiced in a relatively open-ended and nonlinear manner. The varied linguistic capacities for communication at each developmental epoch through childhood and adolescence also represent a barrier to codifying the process. We are accustomed to manualized treatments for specific anxiety disorders, which take the form of sequence-governed programs designed for cognitive-behavioral approaches to therapy. Specific modules of intervention, such as cognitive restructuring and behavioral techniques (e.g., exposure techniques) can be adapted systematically more easily than the open-ended, individualized, and patient-focused narratives that drive the psychodynamic psychotherapy. Similarly, most therapists expect children's ability to attend to rules to be tenuous and erratic. To make the leap to a systematic manualized dynamic treatment, we embrace some of the observational, patient-centered vantage as prescribed by psychoanalysts. Moreover we must listen to and watch the child at play or in conversation to determine our points of entry for intervention without prejudice. We seek openings in natural conversation so that we may approach affect-laden personal stories as they unfold.

We permit the child to present in speech or play in a relatively open manner, watching carefully for what is said, what themes emerge, what symptoms are elaborated, and what his/her attitude is toward the therapy and the therapist. The presenting anxiety symptoms remain the therapist's focus at all times. At the same time we ask the therapist to notice *what is absent,* who is not mentioned, and what seems to be the stance of vigilance and soft spots in the affective vulnerability of the adolescent or child. These observations converge in the therapist's mind into *dominant themes and dynamisms* and focused complaints or disappointments or directed affects such as anger. In the anxious child, central dynamisms revolve around themes that give rise to anxiety.

Unrequited crushes or competitive themes may dominate the stories from life during consultation. Common roles chosen by children of various ages for their therapists may at first blush seem inappropriate after so brief a meeting. These are *displacements from parents or peers* that become obvious to the therapist but remain often unrecognized by the child, but nonetheless seem natural and facilitate the dialogue. Adolescents, especially teenaged girls, impart a chumship role to the therapist at the outset. For latency-aged children the unfair parent or sibling is a frequent mental projection. In younger children the punitive or indulgent projections cast onto the therapist may be most prominent.

Whatever is said or played on then becomes the thematic focus for the next steps in the interventions that will be prescribed only after a set of central dynamisms is uncovered and put into words. Thus, although the steps are not scripted in child and adolescent anxiety psychodynamic psychotherapy (CAPP), the approach is illuminated in this manual, and the path can be cleared of debris and obscuring distractions so that the themes can be brought into the child's awareness relatively rapidly. They can now be witnessed in light of verbal descriptions that can and must be repeatedly revisited in the various and redundant versions of similar stories, with various casts of characters, and in different contexts. These common themes indicate that such situations are associated with the child's anxious, unhappy, depressed moods. Children feel trapped by their experience of the world and its inhabitants in a stereotyped way, imparting a sense of repetition without flexibility or an alternative way out. *This has been called the patient's particular transference pattern (see Glossary), or "role responsiveness," wherein the object of the ire or passion is continuously modeled in a rigid template that is unconsciously stamped onto new and unrelated experiences. It is this inflexible repetitive emotional pattern that the child plays out that the therapy seeks to uncloak and translate into words so that the patient and therapist can look together at the seemingly inevitable constellations of rejection, unwanted attention, or hostility.*

In this mutual quest, it is permissible with younger children to play roles such as detectives or archaeologists or explorers in order to enlist the participant nature of the task of psychotherapy. This new scrutiny seeks alternative meanings to be considered and alternative action patterns that may be possible that will ultimately break the rigid templates that mold expectations in a narrower than necessary constraining interactive constellation. It becomes the task of the therapy to articulate and, later, to break the pattern that had been formulated unconsciously and constructed out of past primitive anxieties and protective defenses. These confrontations with fixed scripts are articulated in words, hopefully to be revised without the associated negative affects. *These repetitive experiences are in fact anachronisms belonging to fantasied themes and constellations, outside of the child's or teen's awareness. The therapy is geared toward unconscious hidden meanings that, when exposed to the light of day and reason, can be studied, understood, and altered. They may then be discarded as intelligible anachronisms or child-like responses to irrational fears.*

This manual articulates therapeutic techniques to focus and place special emphasis on especially anxious themes, whether they emerge in social anxiety and public display or as avoidances or awkward removal from social encounters or unseemly fear and comfort seeking with special persons. The therapist's sequential and directed observations are based on the meanings that the child ascribes to events and incorporates in his/her inner life of personal fantasy as daydreaming and unconscious fantasies. Such unconscious fantasies can be observed by their results in fixed and repetitive maladaptive interactions. The therapist directs his/her attention to verbalizing that which has only been tacitly recognized or is implicit in various action patterns. This focused attention helps the patient recognize the "enemy" in its various guises and in the company of the therapist. The aim is to master rigid response patterns and replace them with more flexible interactions and responses that do not lead to blind tunnels of unhappy repetition.

For example, the child who repeatedly dresses in a manner that suggests babyishness and invites teasing represents a small example of unconsciously promoting attack and feelings and experiences of injustice and passive victimization. To establish this the therapist must first recognize that the patient's protective shields represent various defensive maneuvers, unconsciously set up to manage situations and anxiety as best as they could have been developmentally in the past. Among the most dangerous of these defenses is *projection and denial* because *these defenses tend to distort reality*. The patient does not recognize how his/her beliefs and behavior seem unrealistic because the patient's primary aim is to self-protect from the danger of the internally generated and experienced anxieties and danger situations. These inner demons and fears are generated usually by a *distorted view of frightening fantasies that must be faced*. The stripping of defense is only possible when the patient has a sense of safety and can count on the therapist as a cooperative, friendly adult protector in an imagined inner life of dangers. This cooperative spirit may be temporary as the adolescent seeks autonomy, but *cooperation serves as a way station to autonomy*. The patient, step by step, learns the various forms of dangerous fantasy and its attendant dangerous affects. Gradually, the patient sees the overlap and the pull to regress to old solutions such as clinging to the mother, fearing the shame of exposure, or avoiding peers. The prompts to healthier solutions only become apparent after organizing unconscious fantasies lose their sting and can be reflectively considered.

The focused dynamisms and themes can be recognized in *three or more domains of experience,* in the *anxiety symptoms,* in the *play or transference,* in the patient's *current life,* and from *memories of the past. The more these fantasies are seen to be represented in these domains, the more convincing their evidentiary significance becomes to the patient.* For example the child who has lost a loved one anticipates loss in the present relations as well as loss of the therapist. If the narratives seem salient in so many places, they must be important and very real, even though they are indeed creations of the child's mind. Nonetheless, children do fear harsh teachers, become upset by overprotective parents, and suffer hypochondriac bodily concerns. These concoctions have been cast in the primitive mind of the child and sustained often at least partly unconsciously, and they re-emerge in the more mature child or adolescent who no longer believes in witches, that the mother might eat you, that the father might cut off vital parts, or that a sibling could harm you. These core fantasy structures/terrors are scrutinized in psychotherapy as fossils that no longer carry the same terror and life they once carried, and through reflective revisits these core fantasies are rendered less poignant and salient and, in this way, eventually lose their terrifying meaning. It is in this domain that the work of this manual becomes clear. *The therapist chips away at manifestations of the anxious experience, exposing underlying affective connections and their constricting role in rigidifying new encounters.* The themes gradually are demystified and detoxified. The patient, now less handicapped, is more comfortable to defy the less potent fears and move on his/her own after the therapeutic meetings end.

CAPP differs from more open-ended psychodynamic psychotherapies both in its consistent focus on anxiety symptoms and in its time limitation. The time limitation imparts an urgent, active quality throughout the therapy; when patients have less-communicative sessions, which might not necessarily be addressed in open-ended psychotherapy, the CAPP therapist actively pursues anxiety anyway, as the pressure of termination looms. In a similar vein, the CAPP therapist must always be mindful of the child's reaction to separations even more acutely than in open-ended psychotherapies because the termination date and the child's potential attendant reactions and difficulties must be anticipated. Time limitation is a mobilizing force in CAPP.

Maintaining a dynamic symptom focus probably presents the greatest challenge for experienced psychodynamic clinicians. Anxiety symptoms represent windows into the child's inner life, and uncovering the music and underlying meanings of these symptoms is a crucial element of the way the treatment works to alleviate anxiety. This is approached clinically with careful attention to timing and situations in which anxiety emerges, as well as by pursuing the child's thoughts and feelings during anxiety episodes, which can be explored either verbally or through play themes.

Children and teens often find their anxiety symptoms embarrassing, and it is not uncommon for patients to underreport their self-generated limitations and shameful worries. The embarrassment, or the child's sense of humiliation about his/her symptoms, should be openly noted. Children may label their anxiety symptoms (e.g., phobias, avoidances) with names that feel more acceptable than actually saying the word "fear." They do not wish to seem babyish, younger, and ineffectual rather than as effective and grown-up as their peers.

2.2. Reflective Functioning

There is evidence that improved reflective functioning (RF) and, more specifically, symptom-specific RF mediates the therapeutic interventions and improvement with dynamic psychotherapies (1, 2, 3). RF (Box 2.1) and mentalization are psychological capacities, that refer to the concept of Theory of Mind, which is defined as the ability to attribute mental states, such as beliefs, intents, desires, pretense, and knowledge, to oneself and others and to understand that others have beliefs, desires, and intentions that are different from one's own. RF is a normal cognitive capacity that emerges over the course

---

BOX 2.1 Reflective Functioning

Theory

1. Capacity to think about motivations and feelings in self and others (Theory of Mind)
2. Realization that overt behavior is sometimes regulated and directed by nonconscious thought and fantasy
3. Capacity to recognize patterns of behaviors and associated emotions

Therapy

4. Application of dynamic psychotherapy designed to enhance and use reflective functioning
5. Establishment of anxiety triggers and tolerance of fantasies and conflicting feelings (observing fantasies for their anxious valence)
6. Work toward improving self-observation (a feature of reflective functioning)
7. Cultivation of the recognition and tolerance of anxious experiences associated with fantasies (self-soothing)
8. Attainment of increased flexibility of behavior as intensity of anxiety fades with understanding

---

of early childhood and develops further well into late adolescence and early adulthood (4). Well-developed RF allows individuals not only to understand their own mental states but also to attribute mental states to others. RF comprises self-reflective and interpersonal components. Our definition of RF is largely based on Fonagy, Target, and Steele's (5) definition. There are some variations in regard to the terminology, but RF and mentalization are often used interchangeably. Fonagy and Target describe RF as the "developmental acquisition that permits children to respond not only to another person's *behaviour*, but to the children's *conception* of others' beliefs, feelings, attitudes, desires, hopes, knowledge, imagination, pretense, deceit, intentions, plans and so on" (5, p. 5). This, in turn, allows children to attribute meaning to other peoples' behaviors, thereby making what occurs in relationships understandable rather than apparently random. Fonagy and Target (6) emphasize the interaction between the child's ability to explore and understand the behaviors and actions of others and the growing capacity to "label and find meaningful his own psychic experiences, an ability that we suggest underlies affect regulation, impulse control, self monitoring, and the experience of self-agency" (6, p. 92). They describe this developmental process (i.e., the acquisition of RF) as "the developmental acquisition that permits children to respond not only to another person's behavior, but to the child's conception of others' attitudes, intentions or plans. Mentalization enables children to 'read' other peoples' minds" (p. 92), an ability also referred to as meta-cognition.

Well-developed RF is a normative capacity that helps make behavior in oneself and others intelligible, promotes and maintains attachment security and facilitates recognition of the distinction between real and not-real, hence making the world less frightening. RF enhances communication and encourages meaningful connections between the inner world and outer world. According to Fonagy et al. (5), RF is never fully acquired and typically not maintained in the same way across situations. Individuals differ in their capacity for RF, and there is situational variability even within the same individual.

Mentalizing skills have multiple determinants and develop through interaction with the parent or caretaker. Parents set examples and give feedback to the child, reflecting on their beginning expression of RF. Pretend play allows for integration of inner reality and outer reality, a requisite element of well-developed RF that perforce is related to development of reality testing in children insofar as it must take into account the minds and intentions of others.

Other authors who made a significant contribution to the integration of developmental studies and psychoanalysis are Mayes and Cohen (7). These authors outlined the reciprocal influence of developmental studies of children's developing reflective functioning on psychoanalytic thinking and vice versa. Mayes and Cohen initially detail studies from neuropsychological developmental research, which inform psychoanalytic understanding of the child's growing awareness of his/her own mind as well as others' minds, followed by psychoanalytic observations of early childhood parent-child interactions that show how the emerging understanding of the functioning of their minds is contextualized. The emergence of RF is often dated to the later preschool years, four to six years of age, but the development of RF may be a gradual process and less punctuated. Some authors such as Coates (8) in her comment on Fonagy and Target's 1998 (6) paper postulate that this capacity may start as early as the first months of life with the affective resonance between mother and infant, described by Stern (9). Stern proposes a more advanced quality at the end of the first year of life, when the infant can share a focus of attention with the caregiver and begins to react to meaningful responses the infant has elicited. Such proposals focus on the possibility of intersubjectivity as an anlage for RF rather than an achievement of rational cognition that requires more differentiation and recognition of the mind of another than a communion between mother and infant.

Fonagy and colleagues developed further applications for diagnostic, research, and therapeutic purposes, using the construct of RF. They developed the Reflective Functioning Scale, which is used for diagnostic and research purposes. It is based on Main's (10) Adult Attachment Interview, using memories of individuals, often parents or parents-to-be, of their relationships with their own parents during their childhood. One purpose of the parental Reflective Functioning Scale is that it predicts young children's capacity for RF by their parents' RF.

Fonagy and Target (6) developed a modified psychotherapeutic/psychoanalytic technique for polysymptomatic youth, focusing specifically on enhancing reflective processes. The work does have a strong focus on the affective relationship between patient and therapist in the here and now (6, 8).

Bateman and Fonagy (11) describe difficulties with the mental processes underlying these meta-representations in children and adults with various types of psychopathology, including personality disorders. These individuals have limited reflective abilities, and it is difficult for them to think about their own mental experiences, as well as the meaning of the behaviors of the people with whom they are interacting. Consequently, their responses lack symbolic understanding and flexibility and are often rigid, stereotyped, and nonsymbolic, lacking reflection and modulation.

While the etiology of these developmental disturbances is not known, one hypothesis is that impaired RF in the parent who has difficulties thinking of the meaning of the child's experiences and mind interferes with helping the child build up a "self-structure," which becomes part of his/her sense of self. This creates difficulties for the child to experience thoughts and emotions as originating from within, and the child, in turn, is likely to have insufficiently developed RF capacities, which can lead to developmental personality disturbances (6). One extreme manifestation of this would be in children who suffer abuse and neglect.

Rudden and Milrod (12) further refined the construct of RF by introducing the concept of symptom-specific RF. This was developed in the context of treating adult patients with panic disorder using panic-focused psychodynamic psychotherapy (PFPP), a time-limited psychodynamic psychotherapy approach (13). Rather than having an overall impaired RF capacity, these patients' impairments are organized specifically around their panic symptoms and their emotional significance. Rudden et al. (3) found that symptom (panic)–specific RF improved with PFPP compared with applied relaxation therapy (ART). By understanding the identified central psychological dynamisms surrounding panic and its manifestations during treatment, patients' symptoms improve as the underlying significance of those symptoms becomes more tolerable.

An example of a patient with low RF would be one who expresses certainty rather than doubt over an affectively distressing experience, such as 12-year-old Rob, who states, "I just know that no one ever wants to play me with me," rather than expressing doubt over whether other children would want to play with him and, if not, why that might be and whether he might be contributing something to the situation.

2.3. Case: Seven-Year-Old Miranda

Miranda, a seven-year-old girl with panic disorder, hollered at her therapist that the therapist should not bring up her panic attacks because "It's private!" This patient later compromised with her doctor, permitting discussion about what she labeled "my weirdness."

Almost everything that takes place in these time-limited, anxiety-focused therapies should be viewed as an association to the child's anxiety, in the same way that material presented by patients in more traditional psychoanalytic psychotherapy after they report having a dream can be understood as an association to the dream.

Thus Miranda routinely set up games in the office with her therapist in which she and the therapist played at being co-teachers of a crowd of second-graders, or in which they were pretending to be in charge of an after-school program together. These games were understood by the therapist as representing a *reversal of situations* in which Miranda tended to feel frightened and lost, terrified that she would not understand something important, or in which she might ultimately lose her mother. Timely interpretation of the restitutive function of these games helped Miranda to be less anxious in school.

When Miranda shouted at her therapist that her explosive panic attacks were "private," the therapist asked her why she felt that these events were such secrets, particularly from the therapist.

> THERAPIST: Actually, you come and see me partly because you get so frightened like that, so I'm not sure why it's such a top secret.
> MIRANDA: Because! Mommy's not supposed to tell anyone! I don't like it!
> THERAPIST: Of course you don't like it when that happens, no one likes it when that kind of really scary feeling happens, and I know for you it's very hard to stop the feeling. . . .
> MIRANDA: No, but people think I'm a stupid baby and I hate that anyway because I'm so short (crying).
> THERAPIST: Are you worried that I would think you're a stupid baby?
> MIRANDA: (nods her head vehemently, crying).
> THERAPIST: Oh, I see. You really want me to know what a big, grown-up girl you mostly are, I get it.
> MIRANDA: (cheering up) Yeah, that's it. . . .

The therapist was able to use this observation later in therapy to help Miranda to see patterns that recurred in multiple relationships in her life (with teachers, her father, and a few friends). The simple observation frames Miranda's symptoms developmentally as well, highlighting that they represent something embarrassing and childish to her and emphasizing that she is not entirely as immature as she feels during panic episodes. The idea of embarrassing secrets became an important focus and understanding about her anxiety.

There is a prescribed termination in CAPP in which the child will be expected to resume the next portion of his/her life within the family without the therapy. Autonomy is incipient within the narrow confines of the therapy, but there can be a regression in symptom expression because children often feel abandoned as termination approaches. This dynamism becomes evident in situ and needs to be brought to light and verbalized as a response to the threat of abandonment by the therapist and the frightening feelings that accompany new-found autonomy. In this final burst of emancipation from the therapy, *the drama of attachment and its pull toward dependency is replayed and remastered—this time verbalized rather than just enacted, hopefully as a feature of maturation—not in the paws of servitude to frightening inner voices.*

2.4. Summary

This manual thus contains the skeletal structure of an approach to greater maturity and liberation from childish anxiety. It provides clues and sequences of processes and prompts to therapeutic interventions in designating the anxiety constellations that inhibit developmental progress. It is a guide to healthier development unfettered by rigid containment of all affects in the name of self-protection. Following that, these fantasies are stripped of their magical danger, leaving the inner narrative free of negative and dangerous poignancy aggravated by unconscious fantasy elaboration. The treatment has a structure, and it contains prescribed rules of progress. Thus it is a manual with a beginning, during which the problem is articulated and elaborated in its extent and various forms. During the second phase this elaborated focus is further encouraged and articulated, and the therapist and child review the repetitive aspects of the same dynamisms. Their role in shaping the child's life is highlighted and revisited across experiences in the present, in the past, and in the transference when possible. The termination phase requires preparation for autonomy because the threat of abandonment sometimes revives symptoms that are central in anxiety disorders. All three phases fit together and become coherent and operative for a new beginning with new openness and a greater ability to choose a path.

For those dynamic therapists who believe that therapeutic action is partially, or entirely, in the experience of a new object or the therapeutic alliance or a reworking of earlier psychological relationships, we offer an alternative formulation. The therapy, while interpretive in focus, is also a limited encounter with a more benign and sympathetic coinvestigator/therapist whose time with the patient is briefer, but it certainly comprises new constructive interactional experiences with an adult person who is not a parent.

References

1. Katznelson, H. (2014). Reflective functioning: A review. *Clinical Psychology Review*, *34*(2), 107–117.
2. Kazdin, A. E. (2007). Mediators and mechanisms of change in psychotherapy research. *Annual Review of Clinical Psychology*, *3*, 1–27.
3. Rudden, M. G., Milrod, B., Target, M., Ackerman, S., & Graf, E. (2006). Reflective functioning in panic disorder patients: A pilot study. *Journal of the American Psychoanalytic Association*, *54*(4), 1339–1343.
4. Fonagy, P., Gergely, G., Jurist, E., & Target, M. (2002). *Affect regulation, mentalization and the development of the self*. New York, NY: Other Press.
5. Fonagy, P., Target, M., Steele H., & Steele, M. (1998). *The reflective functioning scale manual* (Version 5).
6. Fonagy, P., & Target, M. (1998). Mentalization and the changing aims of child psychoanalysis. *Psychoanalytic Dialogues*, *8*, 87–114.
7. Mayes, L. C., & Cohen, D. J. (1996). Children's developing theory of mind. *Journal of the American Psychoanalytic Association*, *44*, 117–142.
8. Coates, S. W. (1998). Having a mind of one's own and holding the other in mind: Commentary on paper by Peter Fonagy and Mary Target. *Psychoanalytic Dialogues*, *8*, 115–148.
9. Stern, D. (1985). *The interpersonal world of the infant*. New York, NY: Basic Books.
10. Main, M., & Goldwyn, R. (1994). *Adult attachment rating and classification system* (Manual in draft, Version 6.0). Unpublished Manuscript, University of California at Berkeley.
11. Bateman, A., & Fonagy, P. (2013). Mentalization-based treatment. *Psychoanalytic Inquiry*, *33*(6), 595–613.

12. Rudden, M. G., Milrod, B., Meehan, K. M., & Falkenstrom, F. (2009). Symptom-specific reflective functioning: Incorporating psychoanalytic measures into clinical trials. *Journal of the American Psychoanalytic Association, 57*(6), 1473–1478.

13. Busch, F. N., Milrod, B. L., Singer, M. B., & Aronson, A. C. (2011). *Manual of panic focused psychodynamic psychotherapy—eXtended range*. New York, NY: Routledge.

A Developmental Approach to Children's Communications

A Walk Through the Developmental Stages

3.1. Introduction and Theory

Achieving a therapeutic relationship with a child or teenager depends on embracing a level of comfort with a developmental perspective that respects and encompasses the changing capacities and experiences of children at all stages. The emergence of human autonomy arises from a long process of evolutionary maturation mixed with experience. The process is characterized by progressive age expectations of sequential, behavioral achievements and learning, but is also constrained by built-in limits in biologically determined capacities. Our most distinguished developmental thinkers (Box 3.1) project a progressive timetable that involves maturational opportunities that are influenced by cultural shifts and variability in learning. Piagetian (1) stages are built on such a model, and Vygotsky's "zone of proximal development" (2) projects the emergent next developmental step as a result of the integration of emerging biological readiness and new learning at each successive stage.

Bowlby (3) used a psychoanalytic frame of reference, augmented by ethological models derived from other species, to elaborate the meanings of separation anxiety and its opposite, secure attachment. This is a developmental model of anxiety as a biological survival signal that combines inbuilt readiness to attach as well as adequacy of parenting. He posits species-specific response systems that are awakened by mothering during sensitive periods that become the core of the attachment. Secure attachments are fostered by a dyadic achievement that includes the toddler's sustaining an internal working model of safety and comfort as he/she explores the surrounding environment. As maturation permits, the anxiety aroused by separation is reduced to a "signal," as Freud accurately described it (see Glossary).

BOX 3.1 Developmental Theorists

Ainsworth, Mary, PhD (1913–1999). American-Canadian Professor of Psychology at the University of Virginia. An early collaborator with John Bowlby, responsible for establishing the widely used "Strange Situation" designed to test and designate security of attachment and experimentally validate the Bowlby proposals concerning attachment. **Mary Main** subsequently created the Adult Attachment Interview and its scoring as a further probe in understanding the dyadic nature of the theory.

Bowlby, John, DMP (1907–1990). Psychoanalyst and psychiatrist who broke away from the Kleinian school in London to work for the World Health Organization study of children orphaned by war and then directed the Tavistock Clinic in London. His book, *Maternal Care and Mental Health,* was followed by a three-volume oeuvre, *Attachment and Separation,* elaborating his Attachment Theory derived from an amalgam of Psychoanalytic Theory and Ethology. His close association with Mary Ainsworth secured his place in history by establishing empirical data for his widely acclaimed model.

Bruner, Jerome, PhD (1915–2016). Harvard Professor of Developmental and Educational Psychology and later Oxford Professor who spent his later years at New York University. His broad social and interactive perspective was highly influential in achieving educational developmental models that were socially applied. His later work on the role of narratives was adopted by students of linguistics and literature and further offered a creative approach to meaning in development.

Erikson, Erik S., PhD (1902–1994). Professor at Harvard. Erikson, born in Germany, spent his early years working as an art tutor at a small private school in Vienna, attended by young analysands of Anna Freud. He then moved to the United States and spearheaded Freudian Ego Psychology and developmental theory applied to culture best documented in *Childhood and Society*. His later work in Identity Formation in adolescence rounded out a major creative contribution to principles of development. His ideas concerning identity remain the core framework that helps us understand emergent problems during the reconciliations required for mature behavior.

Fonagy, Peter, PhD (1952–) Hungarian born, United Kingdom–educated psychoanalyst and developmental psychologist. Professor at University College London and Director of Anna Freud Center in London. Fonagy has made major contributions to the articulation of psychoanalytic psychology during the late 20th and recent 21st centuries. He has championed empirical studies of psychoanalytic proposals and directed outcome studies of psychodynamic treatments as well as promoting new models of mentalization-based treatments and studies of reflective functioning. His innovative approaches to treatment have reshaped many of our proposals about the dynamics of borderline personality disorder and anxiety disorders in children.

Freud, Anna (1895–1982). Psychoanalyst. Daughter and significant intellectual and theoretical expander of Sigmund Freud's idea of development who elaborated some of his most cherished programs, the role of defense and compromise in neuroses, and the significance of development and child analysis to our understanding of children. Her model of Developmental Lines remains a clinical masterpiece permitting differential attention to developmental progression rather than symptom and inhibition as pathological focus. Her leadership at the Anna Freud Nursery in London remains an ongoing seat of research and learning.

Kagan, Jerome, PhD (1929–). Professor Emeritus at Harvard and a major contributor to developmental knowledge. Following his PhD he spent a number of years making sense of the data from the Fels longitudinal data, after which he embarked on his own research. He is best known for his work on temperament, focusing on the follow-up of inhibited, shy toddlers and their later appearance at clinic. Their tendency toward anxiety disorders has been verified as a longitudinal outcome from early presentation. His books devoted to developmental theory, including *An Argument for Mind* (Yale University Press), are part of our basic library of developmental understanding.

Mahler, Margaret S., MD (1897–1985). Hungarian-born, German-educated pediatrician and psychoanalyst who emigrated to the United States and worked during her mature years in New York as a child psychoanalyst and researcher who initially studied autistic children and ultimately provided her theory of normal developmental paths in her own Separation Individuation Theory. She directed the Masters Children's Center and team, which included notably Manuel Furer MD, Fred Pine PhD, and Anni Bergman PhD. She has been a major contributor to an ego psychological perspective on development that comprehensively encompasses Attachment Theory.

Piaget, Jean, PhD (1896–1980). A Swiss developmental psychologist who provided a dynamic framework that seriously contested and complemented the behaviorist view of development. His "genetic epistemology," derived originally from observations of his own three children, provided the key steps in our understanding of cognitive development from earliest sensory motor stage to operational abstract intelligence. He is founder of the Geneva school of developmental cognitive studies, and his work continues to challenge more recent nativist developmental theorists.

Stern, Daniel, MD (1934–2012). New York born and bred, he moved from his medical education and psychiatric training to psychoanalysis and took up the challenge of plotting the developmental path in an inclusive manner, including maternal care as a major feature of interactive communication and self-development. He is responsible for microanalytic interactive developmental observations that he used to understand dyadic interactions as development progresses. These observations were applied to adult therapeutic communication as "Now Moments," or "Moments of Meeting." He is responsible for homely developmental designations such as "joint attention" and "social referencing" and stages in self-development.

Vygotsky, Lev S., PhD (1896–1934). A Belarus-born, Soviet-educated developmental psychologist whose careful and cogent observations helped formulate a unique school of developmental psychology that elaborated on Pavlov's early work. He and his student coworker Alexander Luria spearheaded interests in developmental psychology in the Soviet Union, which did not reach the West because of delays in translation until well after the Second World War. He was also a mentor of Urie Bronfenbrenner, who taught developmental psychology from a social perspective at Cornell University. Terms such as "zone of proximal development" highlight the intrinsic organism's readiness to be modified by learning in a systematic progression during development. His untimely death from tuberculosis cut short a most promising career.

Winnicott, Donald, MD (1896–1971). Pediatrician and psychoanalyst. A major figure in psychoanalysis to which he brought an imaginative developmental focus in his large corpus of writing. As a practicing pediatrician who turned to psychoanalysis during the height of Melanie Klein's influence, he modified her views on early development reframing the infant's progression from undifferentiated state to appreciation of those aspects of reality that are salient to progression. His unique homely language remains with us. "Good enough mothering," "there is no such thing as an infant," "transitional object," "the squiggle game" have become part of our popular vocabulary partly because he was enlisted as a BBC discussant at the end of the war years, and mostly because his common-sense language outlasts his sometimes-dense professional texts.

Before Bowlby, Erikson (4) recast developmental stages by adapting Freud's march of infantile experiences as phases and sequences of bodily mastery. Both models thus encompass biological needs experienced as wishes and their counterpart, adaptive compromises, that make up age-related coping as the organism progresses toward maturity. Emotional appeals may become the representations of what Erikson (4) called the "tragedies and comedies that surround the orifices of the body," referring to Freud's body-centered maturational sequence from orality through genital focus as the sites of emotional excitation during the infant's maturation. These elemental, individualized zones are saliently central as parents/caretakers minister to basic biological and emotional needs by caring or, unfortunately, in some cases by lack of caring or even neglect. These foci of body organizational thinking are later stored as bodily preoccupations (embodiments) that are represented as way stations from body to mind, which will be important in symptom formation and, following that, in this therapy. It is only at a later stage of development that these need states represented in mind can be translated to stories of satisfaction and security or deprivation and fear that can be described by the therapist as propositions to be considered by the child: that is, narrative statements, often framed as questions, regarding the child's wishes and experiences of forbidden satisfaction.

More recent literature using the idea of embodiment similarly considers the role of the senses and bodily participation in learning as a vital part of cognition (5, 6, 7). These more recent investigations invoking embodiment as significant features of early learning utilize Vygotsky's (2) observations that at age three, the links between word and thing and word and thought are irrevocable. Nonetheless, the mind's use of this code is only partially secured. Play and other representational media remain important for accessing underlying meanings and distortions, which often form the root of anxiety constellations, which may seem inchoate to our youngest preverbal children. The therapist must keep in mind that play is to be employed as a representation of the thematic preoccupations and unconscious fantasies of the child that perforce relate to his/her anxiety symptoms in this anxiety-focused therapy. The child often experiences dread and anxiety states in general as inchoate, without access to thoughts and words, and it is one of the central roles of the therapist to understand and translate these anxiety preoccupations into words. Play is, thus, a means to crack the code, not an end in itself. The good therapist learns that his/her enjoyments of the play encounters are relationship-building and that the meanings that emerge become the subject for verbalization and reflection as the treatment progresses and reflective functioning becomes empowering.

Acknowledging these stages as changing modes of coping during maturation is essential to making stage-attuned contact with children and adolescents. A simple example derived from language research in early childhood shows that mothers adapt the complexity of use to "motherese," roughly adjusted to a stage above the infants competence, thereby gauging their complexity to the child's developmental capacity to understand. Such adjustment permits attention and better cooperative interaction as well as learning (8).

3.1.1. Preverbal Communication

Infants move away from utter dependency, when caretakers function as the executive who carries out essentials for survival. Human children require buffering and nurturance from outside by a mother/caregiver who permits developmental progress in infant competence with physical and experiential nurture. The mother or other primary caretaker also provides variations in caring and culturally specific practices, dictated by social trends and customs that may change over time. The infant's near-total dependency changes rapidly during the first year of life as the nonverbal child gains some motor control and can sit by six months and stand and then walk between 11 and 18 months. The new possibility for musculoskeletal control permits more finely articulated behaviors such as pointing and designating and the linked ability to express needs by gesture and voice that soon take on an appeal function and permit early gestural-vocal communication as a sign that the other is recognized as a source of satisfaction and soothing.

At about one-year old, this rapidly gives way to phonic vocalizations that become formed words and then early phrases by two-years old that permit proto-play conversations that, from the outside, look like early dialogues, with co-vocalization and later turn-taking. Nonetheless, the preferred gestural communication may also take the form of proto-play, with themes emerging related to the early human interactions (9, 10) that have a role in establishing attachment, a core emotional developmental domain that is found across mammalian species (11). Attachment quality and security can be measured by the Ainsworth Separation-Reunion paradigm between 16 and 22 months (12) based on Bowlby's model. Security of attachment is closely tied to the development of separation anxiety and how and when it is experienced.

Linguists studying infants suggest that the baby is first overheard using expressive utterances initially classified as comfort and discomfort signs (13); later, during the second six months of life, utterances become appeals. Finally, in their most sophisticated forms, utterances become symbolic and can be declarative and propositional (14). In short, motoric and linguistic developmental lines are integrated in a trajectory that permits increasing autonomy as well as increasingly personal and subjective inner thought using a culturally specific language code. This new language acquisition permits and leads to a vertical split between outer speech and dialogue with others and inner fantasy.

3.1.2. Language and Fantasy

Inner dialogue becomes possible because of the human linguistic capacity, and the structured nature of the code provides a vehicle to re-encode unconscious thought/feeling constellations, daydreaming, and fantasy. However, fantasies and daydreams may also take imagistic form and do not always follow the demands of logic. They are a rich store of creative and personal emotionally tinged narratives that may not accede to the logic of linear thought. They are the storybook fairy tales we create to satisfy more than social demands; they are compromises between wish, guilt, and ego demands (15). It is noteworthy that psychophysiological symptoms follow the rules of unconscious thought and fantasy and are emotionally idiosyncratic as well. Fantasies become a lodestone of information regarding a person's inner solutions to complex underlying emotional conflicts and are a child's adaptive means to become comfortable, making compromise solutions and employing defensive actions against fantasized dangers.

Thus, in a seamless way, the toddler engages the world much as Mahler (16) described, in the separation-individuation process. The new capacities of walking and storing organized thoughts are requisite accomplishments for individuation. The toddler can engage in one-to-one encounters or in triadic interactions with the mother and other (e.g., therapist), but the understanding of the therapeutic encounters calls us to accept play, appeal, and gestural behaviors as carrying key content and meaning and to grasp the early personalized speech and language sequences that may require translation from the mother for cogency.

Sometimes, unorthodox personalized "family words" emerge from poor pronunciation or mishearing parents. These neologisms or nonstandard words are responded to in the family and may persist as an intimate home lexicon rather than more common designations of standard language. These personal words become incorporated in the productive vocabulary of the "early linguist." These unique neologisms are frequently affect loaded and carry key interpersonal and familial meanings, which when revived become triggers for more complex affect-laden memories that have been stored and dormant until remembered. Think of a parent of an adult son using such a word in the company of a new girlfriend. The blush of embarrassment is a sign of the secret relationship between mother and son that the word, long out of use, calls to mind.

3.1.3. Development of Separation Anxiety

The emergent representation of the mother in settings of safe early attachment is closely tied to the stranger response at eight months and later separation anxiety that is surely the anlage (origin) for future anxiety experiences, including the extremes of dysphoria seen in anxiety disorders. In normative development "anxiety tolerance" is a developmental landmark that enhances well-being insofar as the exploring curious child learns not to freeze or flee in the face of novelty but rather to explore new experiences. Both Mahler (16) and Bowlby (17) espouse the idea that building a secure attachment involves some internalized positive parenting experiences. This idea is at the root of Bowlby's proposal that the toddler becomes able to use the mother as a safe base from which to explore the world and is therefore adaptive (17). Thus, while early separation anxiety is adaptive, it can become a symptom in later years if the tolerance level associated with separation and autonomy seeking is delayed or poorly developed. The temperamentally shy or inhibited child has a more desperate need to cling and may be more vulnerable to anxiety disorders (26).

Before discussing successive developmental stages and giving concrete examples, we must visit another feature of human cognitive and emotional development—the role of empathy and reflection, which is also discussed in Chapter 2, Section 2.2.

3.1.4. Reflecting on Others

Each of these latter feats requires not only an ample separation of the self from others but also the ability to fancy that other persons also have minds and, when possible, wills that come to be understood as intention as well as another point of view (i.e., Theory of Mind) (18) (Box 3.2). Although there is some evidence that infants during the second half of the first year imitate affects displayed with similar affective states, they are not yet of the same

---

BOX 3.2 Developmental Landmarks Enhancing Reflective Function

- Capacity for interactive play: approximately 1.5 to 2 years on
- Ability to produce a narrative sequence of three steps in speech or play: approximately 2.5 years on
- Ability to think about self and others (Theory of Mind): approximately 3.5 years on
- Evidence of sound short-term memory and ability to reflect: approximately 4 to 5 years on
- Capacity to reflect and take one's thoughts and fantasies as objects for mental consideration (metacognitive function, observing ego): approximately 6 years on

---

structure as empathy when the child can dissociate his/her own self from another and then recognize others' feelings. Those who have studied Theory of Mind in children can show that at about 18 months the toddler can identify the image in the mirror as himself/herself and is capable of separating subjective from objective (19). Other landmarks of import are joint attention, which is social referencing whereby the toddler's eye gaze is directed toward the mother before venturing to do something that has, in the recent past, been interrupted (5). From these early data we infer the ground structure that will become self-reflection and social affects such as pride and shame (19).

This newly learned ability is essential to tolerate taking turns and sharing in nursery school, which require the young thinker to tolerate frustration and interrupt drive expression. These new achievements are also important in psychotherapy in which the therapist taxes the child by referring to others, their wishes, and their intentions. At age six or older, we expect youngsters to reflexively take cognizance of their own actions, stories, and repetitive themes by employing an early maturational form of reflective functioning. We will see how the constraints of language immaturity in children affect referencing and symbolizing but also intertwine with reflection and metacognitive contemplation of self in society (20, 21, 22, 23). Reflective functioning is a postulated mediator of change in open-ended adult "affect focused, including dynamic" therapy (24), and we postulate that Symptom-Specific Reflective Function operates in children who engage in CAPP.

Examples of children's play and dialogue at sequential developmental stages are presented to demonstrate the developmental possibilities and constraints that are associated with the maturing psyche and the available representational possibilities in language at ages two, five, six, 11, and 16.

Although this manual is designed to outline therapeutic interactions with children from ages eight- to 16-years old, these earlier examples of language and conversational competence are included to demonstrate the progressive march from infant dependency, characterized by the absence of language and limited representational capacity to increasing autonomy and the emergence of symbolic referencing in a code. Earlier modes of expression can be observed even among the older age group of children targeted by child and adolescent anxiety psychodynamic psychotherapy (CAPP). Formats for regressive thinking at ages encompassed in CAPP therefore apply in this manual. As a complement to these factors, we must attend also to the environmental strains the child experiences and to the borrowed use of words and phrases taken from parents and the immediate dialogic environment (8).

3.2. The Playing, Dependent Child

3.2.1. Play Psychotherapy Technique With Young Children

During play psychotherapy with young children the "down and dirty floor time" brings the child therapist to eye level with the child and to the interactions carried out on the young child's terms, learning to translate what is communicated in play and reading of themes that emerge from observations (Box 3.3). This requires, as in therapies with older children and adolescents, that the therapist be attentive to *repetitions* and *redundancies* and to *affective accompaniment* and defensive *changes in pace and theme* as well as *breakdowns from formerly fluid action* and coherence in play as signs of distress. These observable "surface" behaviors can be useful in detecting defense and conflict, just as volume and cadence appear as prosody, marking affective valence and urgency of any utterance. Later, fine-motor, articulated control may permit the introduction of pencil-and-paper games and drawings and more therapeutically sophisticated interventions such as the squiggle game (26) by age three, allowing the child to express ideas and feelings with participation of the therapist.

In embarking on a path of any psychotherapy, including psychodynamic psychotherapy, we must form an assessment about the relative autonomy of the child/adolescent as well as his/her communicational competence, comprehension, and capacity for self-awareness and reflective functioning. Children with inhibited temperaments in early childhood are at risk for later frank anxiety disorders that are seen after age seven (26). These factors will necessarily converge to dictate the therapist's choice of means and vehicles of exchange (talk, play games, pretend) and the need for other props (toys or paper and pencil) and even of whether

---

BOX 3.3 Strategies for Working Therapeutically With Play

- Representational narratives include dramatization and pretend roles with toys/dolls or with therapist
- Variation of representational media/toys (examples: drawing, mimicry)
- Attend to thematic coherence, discover commonality
- Verbalize themes and interpretations
- Relate themes to desires, defenses, and meaning of anxiety
- Show relationship of ongoing feelings to anxiety
- Demonstrate repetitions of earlier representations in new media or talk

the parent must be seen with the child and how frequently to arrange meetings. Children of ages two and a half to 10 years may engage in *play* and/or *talk* therapy some or all of the time as long as the vehicle of expression is salient, relevant, and familiar. Permitting the parent to be present in the room during the treatment should not be encouraged, especially in older children, because it reinforces the dependency and diminishes the self-conscious aspect of agency and autonomy that constitute reflective functioning.

The foundational literature in child psychoanalysis, from Hug-Hellmuth (27) and Klein (28) on, describes using play as a substitute for free association to track psychologically recurrent themes and fantasies and preoccupations. The play and its themes and interruptions enable the therapist to follow the flow of unconscious mental narratives and their variations as well as defensive maneuvers that are operative as difficult themes emerge. The particular vehicle of expression and the content of play themes may change even in the microcosm of a single therapeutic session, but the meaning units and narratives that the play represents highlight the salient fantasies that are translated into stories that encode preoccupying unconscious worries and themes.

There are differing technical opinions about whether the thematic material should interpreted in the play alone or whether it should be related to life themes and made explicit and actually generalized for reflective use at a more neutral time, such as during clean-up as the session winds down (29). Whether translated and integrated or not, an aim of therapeutic play in CAPP is to relate the immediate content/themes to the anxiety symptoms and also, less centrally, to the transference as well as to the ongoing dramas in the child's life. Following this path, *a connection to the past is sought to translate the construct of the thematic preoccupation into words that encompass the child's experiences in what will become a discovered coherent story between the therapist and patient and may highlight elements that are less than adaptive or even destructive and contribute to symptoms.* In summary, the organizing theory of CAPP may be stated as follows:

> The play and verbal current presentations represent themes that match unconscious compromises and fantasies that refer to the past and are repeated in life in the present, in symptoms, in relationships external to that with the therapist, and in the transference with the therapist. The focus in CAPP concerns meanings associated with the experience of anxiety, whether elicited by external/social or internal triggers or a sense of unnamed danger.

3.2.2. Case: Normally Developing Two-and-a-Half-Year-Old Mary-Beth

The vignette of Mary Beth at age two and a half is a developmental example of a normal youngster.

Mary Beth was unknowingly observed at solitary play and was overheard in sub-vocal accompaniment to play with her dolls: "Put on her hat (Dolly was unclothed); What's the matter?"; "He's OK honey!"; "Come see my friends"; "This is my mommy "; "I'm going to school"; "I'll come back soon"; "I get dressed". This brief segment reveals a great deal about this child's developmental capacities as well as her preoccupations and the sources of her word use. Clearly Mary-Beth is past the 2-word phrase language structure expected. She is capable of forming designative phrases that are representative of real life events, and she applies them to her play objects. She recognizes the dolly as referencing the human form in fantasied human interactions. The sequences are fragmented, although coherent, and refer to common themes that are elaborated in associated speech - some phrases clearly borrowed from overheard adult speech in her proximal environment.

She uses her own frame of reference and associations to the unclothed doll and, focusing on her nakedness, relates it to Mary-Beth's next task of dressing prior to leaving for imaginary school. This coherent referential sequence invites our curiosity regarding the salience of day-to-day separation from her caretaker, temporary distraction in play as a bridge to reunion, and finally the daily routines of dressing prior to entering a broader outer world in the form of attending school. All are unified by the reassurance that separation is not loss and that return is a vital expectation.

To lend credence to the idea of the intimate relationship between separation from close attachments and anxiety, there is a popular song on a recording for toddlers that reassures by its refrain: "Your mommy comes back, Your mommy comes back. She never will forget you!"

Clearly, the chosen play themes are drawn from salient events in the young child's life, and more important, her wish to replay them in her personal and unique shuffling of stories representing her version of experience encoded in language. Therapies draw on those selected meaningful dramatizations and provide a means of validating the child's experience by encoding them in words.

3.2.3. Case: Five-Year-Old Emily

An encounter with a shy five-year-old Emily is described by Shapiro (30), who employed the Winnicott Squiggle drawing game (25) to become engaged during a consultation for anxiety and sleeplessness that occurred with the deaths of relatives. Briefly, the child's family had recently heard about a distant cousin who tragically died along with two of her three children in a country house fire during the night. The child's symptoms flared after this event. Emily's father was a surgeon, and she was cognizant that he put people to sleep to remove "bumps."

The child clung to her father, and the therapist could not initially separate them. The therapist took out a stack of paper and two pencils, drew some sequential "squiggles," and asked Emily to complete the pictures. Her initial drawings were difficult to decipher without dialogue, but after the third or fourth squiggle, which she only named simply, she was comfortable enough to permit her father to exit the office, and she began to explain what she drew. The length of the session proved to be sufficient to elicit a series of themes that were related to her fear of death if she were to go to sleep, in accord with the story of the fire. The clear leitmotif of being put to sleep to be operated on, as she took on the roles of both nurse assistant to her surgeon father and patient to be subject to "a bump" removal, was evident. For this five-year old, a conscious concern was linked in her mind to personal familial themes of being a grown-up in the role of assistant to her surgeon father coupled with her interpretation of what surgeons remove during sleep. She then commented on her pet guinea pig who was discovered quiet in his cage one morning and then declared dead by her father. The therapist simply noted, "it may be confusing to you because sleeping and dying seem alike, but they are very different and grown ups can tell one from the other without confusion." The therapist further included Emily's fear of death or harm coming to her if she were to fall asleep and linked this to her insomnia and anxiety. The girl's symptoms quickly resolved. While the therapist did not directly translate his full surmise of the theme of her anxiety, he did link the anxiety about sleep to the bad things that she worried could happen while asleep when no one was on guard. In this instance the interpretations were in fact educative and permitted unlinking misbeliefs from a frightening amalgam of co-occurring fantasies.

3.3. The Talking, Autonomous Child

3.3.1. Psychotherapy Technique With School-Aged Children

School-aged children have achieved full locomotion, can physically separate from their parents, and have the fullest skills of language so that they can request, demand, propose, declare, and make propositions about their environment and spin narratives about their inner conscious fantasy life. They can refer to their past wishes about the future. They have recently acquired a more solid moral code and can be judgmental about their caretakers and pay attention to their peers and seek their approval. These achievements of individuation permit relative autonomy, and most primary school systems use six years as the age for schooling, bargaining for what Erikson (31) has designated the "age of industry." These children, however, are dependent on their parents emotionally and for shelter and food, and they are culturally bound to home until the biological signals of puberty encroach on body and mind to set the youth tentatively on a more realistic quest for autonomy, followed by pairing and possibly procreation (21).

Children of this level of developmental accomplishment can engage a therapist in verbal dialogue and can be encouraged to *reflect on their own mind and that of others* (32) and to grasp the differences between nonverbal fantasy, wishes, dreams, and reality, and they can maintain an inner life that represents both verbal and nonverbal images. *They are thus ready for an intervention that employs talk and reflection with relative separateness from parents.*

The experiences of six- and seven-year olds with talking to adults vary, and early therapeutic meetings have to be titrated in a nonthreatening way, shaping queries by the therapist that do not irritate or tax. The therapist's openness should be modulated to fit the child without condescension or arrogance. The shy, slow-to-warm-up child must be permitted easy entry, while the aggressive, impulsive child should not be counterpunched and treated like a "wise guy." Drawing and talking with one another or limited use of board games can help to break the ice. Dollhouses are permitted but are not essential. Most important, the school-aged child's skills for communication are well formed, and talk works at both ends, receptively and expressively. Thus the beginning stages of a therapeutic encounter require tact in accord with the child's character, and the stories that are discovered should be permitted to emerge, rather than being extracted like a rotten tooth or judged. Following general rules of tact, the latency child is ready to participate verbally in a dialogue and to play. The latter can often be suspended as meetings continue. The latency or school-aged child can be a pleasure to work with and provides a genuine coexplorer with an alert therapist, who permissively should allow the unfolding of themes and stories that can be put into words and reorganized with a focus on their relationship to anxiety symptoms, maladaptations, and symbols of skewed relationships and with a readiness for distortions that can be recognized.

When the therapist has obeyed these developmental guideposts, he/she can proceed in uncovering, exposing and confronting anxiety symptoms.

3.3.2. Case: Seven-Year-Old Alice

The bookmaking described next in the case of seven-year-old Alice illustrates one model within the developmental path. Alice was the younger of two adopted children and was brought to therapy for anxiety and temper outbursts. She was reluctant to address the themes and parental issues that led to her referral for treatment. After a number of play opportunities, Alice decided to *draw a book* and asked the therapist to write her dictated text to accompany the pictures. Not by chance, the story was displaced onto a bunny, as in so many of the books commonly read to toddlers, such as the *Runaway Bunny,* Br'er Rabbit stories, and Winnie the Pooh stories. The form of the story, too, had many references to culturally available themes derived from fairy tales such as "Red Riding Hood" and "Hänsel and Gretel." Most important, we did not have to address directly the central theme of her life, her adoption, which would likely have felt like an intrusion. Instead, she embedded her life drama into a complex story and revealed her inner concerns in a tale about leaving home, bewilderment, sense of loss and reunion with a grandparent, and a new addition of a partner, with whom she built a new house and reserved a room for the lost, and then found, granny. The explicit references to adoption indicated from a developmental vantage that her preoccupying worries were translated into working stories that could be approached in the therapeutic encounter to work through the worries, attachments, and wishes that besieged her. "You have now found your grandma and feel safe. By giving her a place to stay with you, you can stop worrying about being lost."

Alice's unwillingness to approach the issues directly suggested that even at age seven she employed defenses that had to be understood as some inner recognition and understanding that her mind was compartmentalized into fantasy and reality elements and that the former may have been embedded in guilt or shame or just a sense of personal privacy, making the themes less open to scrutiny. Without ceremony the therapist's permission to play, draw, and tell her story displaced onto a bunny family, Alice might not have opened the gates that enclosed her personal worries, but this allowed a new grasp of her anxiety and permitted its translation to words.

3.4. The Preteen and Adolescent Youth

3.4.1. Psychotherapy Technique With (Pre) Teen Youth

The hormonal surge that heralds puberty has its dual thrust in both bodily changes and radical cognitive alterations. At the same time, it is cultural adaptations to industrialization and economic changes that have created what is known as adolescence. Adolescence, or what Erikson (31) referred to as a *moratorium,* is the prolonged wait between the initial physical maturational ability to procreate and later engagement in the roles of the adult in the modern cultural community. Across multiple domains and expectations, we can observe that the long gap between biological ability and social readiness has continued to lengthen since the beginning of the industrial revolution.

During adolescence, various tasks and integrations must be accomplished: adaptation to one's own body; adoption of a gender role and sexual identity; de-idealization of one's parents and the adoption of a work path and adult identity; achievement of various forms of personal closeness, chums, groups, and partners; integration of sexuality and intimacy. These are fragmented for discussion but cohere as a developmental unity as teenagers consolidate an identity and personality and move away from home, reaching for a peer community and future means to add to life's cycle by procreating and raising a next generation.

Working with adolescents psychotherapeutically when dependence is giving way to autonomy requires some adjustments in therapist stance. The therapeutic encounter during this stage is not easily approached unless the therapist can tap his/her own adolescent memories and find distance from the grown-up parental role, enabling management of the clear split between the aims of parents and the unique but conflicted aims of adolescents. Anna Freud's description of therapeutic neutrality (32) can be extended in this instance to seeking equidistance between the adolescent's often ambivalent autonomy seeking and parents' reality-based wishes for safe passage, simultaneous with the inadvertent, mixed pull of dependency and ambivalence.

Adolescents in contemporary Western culture are embedded in a subculture that is marked by rapidly switching dialect that has a specialized, cherished vocabulary, that essentially communicates suspicion of the "grown-up" probes and prying as we attempt to engage as therapists (33). Therapists should not ape/play "the adolescent" in dress or in language because this offends and is insensitive to these peer-group forces. It is important to ask for definitions of what may be seem to be familiar words because meanings rapidly alter over time and current nuances evolve quickly. Some examples are *gender* (verb), *meme, trolling,* and *larping,* but by this week the drift in meanings may be large. During the current computer age the changes in nuance and meaning are even more rapid. When permitted to engage in the peer language code, the next code to grasp is the teenager's personal historical lexicon, which is enmeshed in episodic memory as outlined, personal fantasy, and a sense of self and belonging. For our entire lives we are split between at least two modes of thought, divided between conscious outer-directed speech and effort. Inner personal fantasies comprise ongoing commentaries and compromises on outer and inner experiences. These thought patterns are not unconscious portions of mentation that underlie the structure of our experience but rather emerge as the stories generated during latency and adolescence. They are inner, often compelling, musings and story lines. They are also likely to appear in daydreams, inner deliberations, obsessions, and conscious fantasy.

The adolescent may be emotionally labile and project a sense of fragility. Yet relationships are sometimes short lived and briefly mourned. Yesterday's best beau may be submerged before one can learn the name of the new incarnation of earlier homegrown figures in the latest iteration of a romantic partner.

The new interpersonal relationship with the therapist must be friendly and receptive, but the therapist is not a "friend," nor is he/she a parent or teacher. It is the therapist's receptivity and nonjudgmental stance that will serve as a scaffold on which the adolescent can venture a relationship. This demands authenticity and genuine warmth without the potential to suffocate or join the kids. In that sense the developmental function of the peer chum supersedes that of the guardian, educator, and parent. Adolescents put their therapists on trial and challenge them before they permit a solid trusting dialogue. In this time-limited psychotherapy, time is not on your side, yet more time is available than may initially appear evident. Adolescents don't warm quickly, and once warmed, they do not let go easily, especially when they have entered the encounter with anxiety. Nonetheless, understanding and the feeling of being understood go a long way toward being able to do the work involved in an anxiety-focused psychodynamic treatment.

The therapeutic relationship with an adolescent demands flexible roles. It can at times take on characteristics of a chumship, or peer confidant. At other times the therapist may be cast in the role of a parenting and guidance-offering big sibling, and at still other times like a builder of self-esteem in the midst of a threadbare or absent parental and peer cheering section.

The latter shifting roles may seem tentative at first, and at other times brittle and uncertain. The more the adolescent is in the throes of identity shifts, the greater the therapist must take his/her distance so that the power of the transference is not interpreted as coercion. At times, facing realities about danger becomes central, especially when avoidance leads to school failure. Dependency is still real during adolescence because of the intrinsic struggle for independence during this epoch. The therapist must help the adolescent to tease his/her own personal emerging interests from the parents' attempts to offer advice that is too often unwelcome or frightening because a conflict is set up that confuses the adolescent regarding the origin of the plan—parents or self. A dilemma arises when the adolescent must swallow hard when realizing that his/her own best interests are served and can be autonomously pursued despite agreement with parental opinion. In short, it is OK to do what one's parents advise, and sometimes these aims also foster the adolescent's own cause. Nay-saying to parents can be tic-like and not rationally considered to advance the avowed self-determination. Anxiety is frequently stimulated by the idea that teens are defying parental authority, and they tend to resent the sense that they are being infantilized. Often the core conflicts uncovered in psychotherapy concern the teenager's relationship to work and school, sexuality, intimacy, and life goals. All are of great consequence to the adolescent, but the common sense of urgency, particularly among anxious teenagers, can be distracting and/or overwhelming for therapists. New developmental achievements become muddled by prior childish fantasies and mental solutions that belong to the past. These must be disengaged from childhood solutions that are no longer relevant. Anxiety symptoms serve as sentinel guideposts to these changes, which seem desirable but threaten some of the comforts of still being a child and needing protection.

The therapist, at this developmental crossroad, must be engaged but cognizant of the unevenness of this developmental path. Core conflicts that emerge as the anxiety is unmasked must be highlighted and articulated to be studied and discussed together for better understanding of ways in which maladaptive solutions were established and may no longer suffice. Sources of anxiety in adolescence frequently concern the following matters: fear about separation and security as teens ready themselves to leave the nest; fear of their own anger at hovering parents, yet sometimes greater comfort with rage than an uncomfortable sense of closeness; confusion regarding bodily urges, dealt with by making mental solutions in their sexuality with fantasies secretly satisfied in masturbation; and shame and self-punishment related to the desire to join in reveling with peers, which is seen as "bad."

The therapeutic task with anxious adolescents is to open new possibilities and to broaden the teenager's scope of action and mastery of new relationships by engaging the underlying fantasies that lead to conflict and defense and a narrowed field of action because of inhibition (34).

During this cybercentury with its focus on apps and videogames, the adolescent's selection of wished-for qualities may surface in the avatars chosen while playing these games (35). The desirability relates to a central issue of adolescent life. Budding sexuality can be linked to many exciting but anxiety-provoking themes. How does the teen accommodate to his/her new body, and how does the teen meet the challenge of sexual arousal and whatever changing taboos remain salient in the community? As therapists, we are aware that masturbation and fantasies that come to constitute the conditions for arousal have been cultivated, under ordinary circumstances, in privacy during prior stages of life and may take many forms that seek expression during the teen years in the teen's body and the various fantasies that prompt arousal. Sexting may initiate a private encounter but remains very far from mature intimacy (36). The modern world presents other dilemmas for the therapist of adolescents that pertain to public health issues and adult guidance toward responsible action, such as contraception, safe sex, alcohol and drug abuse, and driving while under the influence. These are clearly family and parental responsibilities but may inadvertently enter the therapeutic dialogue and create problems about how they are to be addressed. Insofar as the adolescent may confess some of these matters, it can be antitherapeutic to take on a parental role of judging the action. Nonetheless, as health-care providers, it is important to handle these—often life and death—topics clearly and openly, taking a no-nonsense, public health awareness approach: unsafe sex, importantly, can lead to transmission of chronic and fatal illnesses, and drugs or drinking and driving are dangerous in reality.

3.4.2. Case: Eleven-Year-Old Preteen Grace

The following case refers to an acute exacerbation of separation anxiety that was experienced by an almost teen as a rejection and abandonment and preference for a rival by a parent and highlights the conflict-laden interplay between autonomy seeking and dependency needs.

Grace, an 11-year-old girl who had a long-standing anxiety disorder with early clinging and repeated episodes of camp refusal, was successful at a two-week sleep-away camp during the past summer, peppered with frequent phone calls to her widowed mother. Her father died three years before after a three-year illness. For the coming summer she asked to try another specialty camp for a week and eagerly approached the grounds with her mother and her mother's boyfriend of the past year. The couple was planning to go on a holiday of their own after delivering Grace to camp. At the opening ceremony Grace bolted and cried unconsolably, and her mother was forced to take her home, defeated by Grace's acute panic attack.

Grace was seen in psychiatric consultation the next week and told her story in the following manner: "My mother wanted me to go to camp because she thought it would be good for me. She thought I had done it last year so I would be able to do it again and it would be something I could be proud of myself for." The therapist noted that that was her mother's story, but he asked Grace what her view of the matter was. She quickly noted with some embarrassment that her mother wanted her away because she was a bother and that her mother would have welcomed some free time alone with her boyfriend. Only at the end of the meeting did the therapist ask Grace what she would like to happen if all of her wishes could be granted. Grace did not hesitate to say that she wished her father were alive. This dialogue must be looked at as a narrative emerging as a coherent story made up of separate parts that were delivered over the time of the interview and that provided explicit links to the underlying meaning of her anxiety symptoms. The preadolescent's story emerged when given tacit permission and time to say what was on her mind, and the therapist's queries did not bind her to a determined sequence. Instead, what emerged was her affectively charged attachment to her mother as well as her veiled anger and worry that her mother was willing to abandon her by choosing her boyfriend over herself in a setting in which she acutely felt the loss of her father anew, and her heightened sense of abandonment and accompanied anxiety was doubled at the thought of loss of her mother.

The storyline and defenses were easily discovered in the dialogue as a whole in this child of 11 who had good social awareness and also anxieties that were driven by wishes and concerns that felt unacceptable to her because in a unique way the wish that her father were still alive was a potential threat to her relationship with her mother, instituting her panic experience at separation. Furthermore, from her perspective, her mother's attachment to her new male friend offered an additional threat to her comfort in dependency because she was being sent off and her mother was selecting someone else. The story also indicates Grace's dependent regression in the setting of the acute separation, as her mother was to leave and choose another rather than her. She panicked, feeling again, as of old, that she still required her mother to buffer her in this test of separation. In addition she could not fully make her wish conscious that her father were alive. Despite excellent adaptive skills and prior age-appropriate social and academic skills, Grace was caught in her revived past that played a role in her panic.

3.4.3. Case: Sixteen-Year-Old Teen Laura

The case of Laura, aged 16, illustrates some of these issues and permits us to recognize the capacity of an adolescent to construct a complex narrative in her own words as the therapeutic relationship proceeds and trust is established, even within the limited time frame of CAPP. Laura lived with her physically sick but functioning mother and 12-year-old brother. Her father was taken ill and died suddenly during the night when Laura was 12, and her mother enlisted her in helping to care for her younger brother. The night of her father's death, Laura stayed home with her brother while her mother joined EMS in transporting her father to the hospital, where he died. The elements of traumatic loss added to this otherwise competent youngster's early separation anxiety. Laura entered psychotherapy with multiple symptoms of anxiety. She was unable to sleep alone and so slept with her mother in her bed every night. She had fantasies of her mother dying when her mother was out late, causing a pattern of anxious waiting. Laura had frequent arguments with her mother about her mother's going out late, and she began to despair that she would never be able to leave home to go away to college on her own, while at the same time, a part of her longed to do so. She longed for independence and resented the added burden of needing to be a substitute caretaker for her brother, yet she also clung ambivalently to her mother.

In therapy, she quickly uncovered her suppressed rage at her mother. Laura secretly had wished it had been her mother rather than father who died. She sorely resented the parentified role she felt stuck in. Aggravating this plight, she feared her mother would die of her illness without her care, and her guilt added to her distress. Laura had sufficient expressive ability to describe her fantasies as well as the multiple strains of meaning around her very mixed, guilt-producing feelings. She recognized that her anxiety functioned to short-circuit her anger at her mother, which felt too dangerous to acknowledge or express. Autonomy and escape from home did not feel like an acceptable goal, so she found herself downplaying her competence and accentuating her weakness with her anxiety.

Laura's budding sexuality was recognized in another compartmentalized set of anxiety symptoms, expressed as a fear of showering if no one was home. She fantasized a break-in while she was in the shower as she imagined someone uninvited observing her nude body. Thus her anxiety symptoms encompassed both aggressive and sexual fantasies about which she had very mixed feelings and protected her from seeking their expression in life. These constellations were placed into narratives in therapy and were the topics of the dialogue between Laura and her therapist. There were opportunities to see the displaced themes in the transference because of her developmental competence. The therapist approached her defensiveness about exposing these thoughts to him as a way of acknowledging that the fantasy of being looked at naked was arousing and frightening at the same time.

The scope of any psychodynamic psychotherapy is always embedded in the developmental principles outlined here because everyone, regardless of chronological age, is always in the flux of incorporating new experiences into old, prior established ways of thinking, established out of conflicts and emotional constraints from the personal past. It is the relative rigidity of these structures based on old narratives that newly create anxiety in the developing teenager and also inhibit new actions and adventures. The therapist must be constantly vigilant so that the ongoing therapeutic relationship does not succumb to the pressure to re-enact past conflicted attachments. This is one reason that the therapist seeks to grasp these past conflicts. The therapist's countertransference, or response to the patient's anxiety and the expectations he/she (often unconsciously) brings to the therapeutic relationship, must be monitored throughout the treatment, as well as the patient's propensity to re-create in the therapeutic relationship a re-enacted role from past core attachments that skews the interaction.

It is important to address Vygotsky's zone of proximal development (2) in treating adolescents; that is, the patient is developmentally close to the time when the next step can be mastered. This allows for the growing person to feel connected to what transpires in treatment, and the patient is not turned off or left with the feeling that he/she is hopeless and that therapy is irrelevant. The therapist in this sense must be a vigilant and thorough student of development and also a connoisseur of the range of human variation and unique social media opportunities available in the modern experiences of the anxious adolescent.

3.5. Summary

Any therapeutic approach to children and adolescents must take into account the capabilities and vicissitudes of the stage of maturation and development of the patient. These considerations make explicit the often rapidly changing role of parents and of growing personal agency, as well as the necessarily central dependency-autonomy struggle of the growing person. This psychodynamic psychotherapy manual, focused on treatment of child and adolescent anxiety, is specifically geared toward such considerations and the parallel changing inner environment and fantasies, stage-related conflicts, defenses, and coping capacities. The therapist has an added burden in his/her relationship to children at various ages and stages, needing to develop some proficiency in recognizing these stages. Child and teenaged patients may parallel the therapist's own children's ages and problems. This makes for dilemmas around countertransference, rearing philosophies, and the new aspects of culture as well as the specific culture of the child in treatment. In this era of cyberspace and smartphones, children can feel constantly observed, too close by a ring of the cellphone and never free of parental vigilance. We have not yet adequately appraised the consequences of such cultural changes on frustration tolerance (of both parents and children) and the ability to tolerate separateness, both qualities necessary for autonomous maturation (36).

References

1. Piaget, J. (1955). *The language and thought of the child.* Cleveland, OH: World Publishing (Original work published 1923).

2. Vygotsky, L. S. (1986). *Thought and language.* Cambridge, MA: MIT Press (Original work published 1934).

3. Bowlby, J. (1958). The nature of the child's tie to his mother. *International Journal of Psychoanalysis, 39,* 350–373.

4. Erikson, E. H. (1963). *Childhood and society* (2nd ed.). New York, NY: W. W. Norton.

5. Stern, D. (1985). *The interpersonal world of the infant.* New York, NY: Basic Books.

6. Fonagy, P., Target, M., Steele H., & Steele, M. (1998). *The reflective functioning scale manual* (Version 5).

7. Fonagy, P., & Target, M. (2007). The rooting of the mind in the body: New links between attachment theory and psychoanalytic thought. *Journal of the American Psychoanalytic Association, 55,* 411–456.

8. Shapiro, T. (1979). *Clinical psycholinguistics.* New York, NY: Plenum Press.

9. Nelson, K. (1989). Monologues in the crib. In: K. Nelson (Ed.), *Narratives from the crib* (pp. 2–23). Cambridge, MA: Harvard University Press.

10. Ninio, A., & Bruner, J. (1978). The achievement and antecedents of labeling. *Journal of Child Language, 5,* 1–15.

11. Milrod, B., Markowitz, J., Gerber, A. J., Cyranowski, J., Altemus, M., Shapiro, T., . . . Glatt, C. (2014). Childhood separation anxiety and the pathogenesis and treatment of adult anxiety. *American Journal of Psychiatry, 171,* 34–43.

12. Ainsworth, M., Blehar, M., & Waters, E. (1978). *Patterns of attachment.* Hillsdale, NJ: Erlbaum.

13. Lewis, M. M. (1936). *Infant speech.* New York, NY: Harcourt Brace.

14. Bühler, K. (1931). *Sprachtheorie.* Jena, Germany: Fischer Verlag.

15. Freud, S. (1911). *Formulations on the two principles of mental functioning* (Standard ed. 12, pp. 213–226). London, UK: Hogarth Press.

16. Mahler, M. S., Pine, F., & Bergman, A. (1975). *The psychological birth of the human infant.* New York, NY: Basic Books.

17. Bowlby, J. (1963). *Attachment and loss: Vol. 1. Attachment.* New York, NY: Basic Books.

18. Bretherton, I. (1991). Intentional communication in the development of an understanding of mind. In D. Frye & C. Moore (Eds.), *Children's theory of mind: Mental states and social understanding* (pp. 271–289). Hillside, NJ: Erlbaum.

19. Lewis, M., Sullivan, M. W., Stanger, C., & Weiss, M. (1989). Self development and self conscious emotions. *Child Development, 60*(1), 146–156.

20. Shapiro, T., & Hertzig, M. (2003). Normal child and adolescent development. In R. E. Hales & S. C. Yudofsky (Eds.), *The American Psychiatric Publishing textbook of psychiatry* 3ed(pp. 67–105). Washington, DC: American Psychiatric Publishing.

21. Shapiro, T., & Perry, R. (1976). Latency revisited, age seven plus or minus one. *Psychoanalytic Study of the Child, 31,* 79–105.

22. Shapiro, T. (2003). Diagnosis and diagnostic formulation. In J. Wiener (Ed.), *Textbook of child and adolescent psychiatry* (2nd ed.). Washington, DC: American Psychiatric Publishing.

23. Shapiro, T., & Amso, D. (2008). School age development. In A. Tasman, J. Kay, J. A. Lieberman, M. B. First, & M. Maj (Eds.), *Psychiatry* (3rd ed., Vol. 1). Philadelphia, PA: W. B. Saunders.

24. Rudden, M. (2017). Reflective functioning and symptom specific reflective functioning: Moderators or mediators? *Psychoanalytic Inquiry, 37*(3), 129–139.

25. Winnicott, D. W. (1971). *Therapeutic consultations with children.* New York, NY: Basic Books.

26. Kagan, J., & Snidman, N. (2004). *The long shadow of temperament.* Cambridge, MA: Belknap Press of Harvard University.

27. Hug-Hellmuth, H. V. (1921). On the technique of child analysis. *International Journal of Psychoanalysis, 2,* 287–296.

28. Klein, M. (1926). Infant psychoanalysis. *International Journal of Psychoanalysis, 7,* 31–50.

29. In-Albon, T., & Schneider, S. (2007). Psychotherapy of childhood anxiety disorders: A metaanalysis. *Psychotherapy and Psychosomatics, 76*(1), 15–24.

30. Shapiro, T. (1983). The unconscious still occupies us. *Psychoanalytic Study of the Child, 28,* 547–567.

31. Erikson, E. H. (1971). *Identity, youth and crisis.* Stockbridge, MA: Austen Riggs Monographs.

32. Freud, A. (1946). *The ego and the mechanisms of defense.* New York, NY: International Universities Press (Originally published in 1936).

33. Shapiro, T. (1985). Adolescent language: Its use for diagnosis, group identity, values, and treatment. In M. Sugar (Ed.), *Adolescent psychiatry* (pp. 297–311). Chicago, IL: Chicago University Press.

34. Freud, S. (1926). *Inhibitions, symptoms and anxiety* (Standard ed. 20, pp. 75–176). London, UK: Hogarth Press.

35. Dreier, M., Wölfling, K., Duven, E., Giralt, S., Beutel, M. E., & Müller, K. W. (2017). About addicted whales, at risk dolphins, and healthy minnows: Monetarization design and Internet gaming. *Addictive Behaviors, 64,* 328–333.

36. Shapiro, T. (2010). *Teen communication.* The Kenworthy Swift Foundation Michael Kalogerakis Memorial Lecture.

4

The Three Phases of CAPP

Opening, Middle, and Termination Phases

This chapter outlines the opening, middle, and termination phases of child and adolescent anxiety psychodynamic psychotherapy (CAPP). The reader is referred to Box 4.1, Therapeutic Process and Strategies, and Box 4.2, CAPP Road Map, throughout this chapter.

4.1. Beginning Therapy: CAPP Opening Phase

4.1.1. Introduction

This initial stage is devoted to a careful assessment of the associations and memories and current behaviors that make up the dynamisms of the anxiety symptoms. The dynamisms are then formulated in words that are used as a focus for the work that follows in therapy. The quest for the underlying meanings of anxiety symptoms and their emotional symbolism requires a careful exploration of the context of targeted symptoms and thoughts as well as inquiry into the origins and timing of the experiences, such as their acuity, chronicity, and the social environment in which they occur. This approach requires listening to the dialogue and/or observing the play at multiple layers from surface to the shadow narrative (1). The shadow narrative is the story that is understood by the therapist just behind the surface, derived with little effort from the words, context, redundancies, and thematic persistence. It also includes the storyteller's persistent tropes and apologies and qualifiers as well as the hesitancies and revisions in midstream that make up the telling itself. We offer a brief play episode of a six-year-old's eagerly repeated surface play in which the racing cars, which he so much loved, could fly and beat everyone, but regrettably had little stopping power or effective brakes. This story's surface narrative was not far from his inner convictions about his wished-for prowess and super powers, but it also said a great deal about his fears about his lack of control and feared recklessness.

BOX 4.1 Therapeutic Process and Strategies

Opening Phase

- History from parents
- Patient developing alliance as narrative of symptoms unfolds in context of life events
- Therapist listening—constructs a dynamic formulation of anxiety symptoms that is shared early-by session 4
  - Primary dynamism identified and presented to child in understandable, experience-near language
- Present dynamism to patient focusing on salience of continuing dialogue where it fits
- Modifying formulation as further information unfolds about meanings of anxiety

Middle Phase

- Continue dialogue—patient begins sessions, sets focus
- Therapist finds recurrent expositions and applies dynamic focus on anxiety
- Patient sharpens capacity to be reflective and self-observing
- Loosening of rigidity of reaction patterns and expanding experiences
- Patient considers other examples in various areas of life of how dynamisms effect anxiety/behavior
- Therapist reinforces reflective functioning (RF) by highlighting recurrent evidence of its use; discusses how improvements in RF temper anxiety and broaden choices

Termination Phase

- Potential symptom rearousal as termination approaches
- Demonstration of transference as focus of anxiety recurrence and separation from therapist
- Repetition and working through dynamisms discovered
- Reinforce reflection and new flexibility of response
- Encouraging new venturesome behavior, demonstrating how using RF can make life less rigid and anxious.
- Revisiting with parents with younger patients and as needed with adolescents

---

The developmental stage and relative immaturity of the patients inform the therapeutic stance toward the child. Younger children may be emotionally engaged and addressed through play and drawing as well as with dialogue, as incidents and stories are gathered for a condensed formulation derived from repeating themes and associated memories and also from vital omissions or breaks in the flow of play or stories as they unfold that

---

BOX 4.2 CAPP Road Map

1. Let patient narrative unfold
2. Listen for associations, omissions, themes
3. Point these out to patient and actively seek clarification
4. Formulate tentative dynamism that underlies anxiety
5. State formulation in words and allow responses that help tailor a better fit
6. The formulated dynamisms of anxiety are subject to change with further information/elaboration ("dynamic")
7. Continue to listen for redundant themes; reinterpret the anxious themes
8. Recast formulation in regard to:
   - External experiences
   - Past experiences
   - Preoccupying symptoms of anxiety
   - Transference examples
9. Encourage self-reflection of repetitive themes (improving symptom-specific reflective functioning)
10. Reinforce observation of return to past dynamisms

---

indicate defenses. We borrow the approach articulated in the Adult Attachment Interview (2), in which grammatical shifts, qualifiers, and other linguistic devices mark the intent of the speaker to bolster our full description of the presentation. The aim of these early interventions is designed to permit a sense of friendly understanding while not presuming to become a peer or an intruder. We permit the stories to unfold and a narrative to develop at a comfortable but steady pace, in a climate of empathic and respectful listening. "Fact finding" in short bursts of questions and answers is to be avoided. The approach is consonant with more open-ended listening utilizing probes, clarification, and contextual elaboration when there is a lack of clarity.

In anxious children, the therapist should not be surprised by the relative lack of autonomy seeking and willingness to seek help. These children are suffering from anxiety and are subjectively in pain, which they recognize in some ways represents their compromised expected autonomy. In many instances, their experience seems natural and ordinary. Thus they are held in mind with little distance from their sense of compromised competence and marred adaptive function. Their neediness is part of their symptomatic experience and contains regressive elements, even if they do not easily admit it. Some of the most fragile of our anxious children externalize their problems defensively by aggressively blaming their parents even as they seem shy and removed at school.

The aim of this initial inquiry will be to create an *organized provisional dynamic formulation* that separates out and names the dominant conflicts and preoccupations of the child and adolescent in a concise, meaningful statement. This working brief narrative is not to be treated as fixed, and it will be subject to editing as therapy progresses. It is a *tentatively held entrée to the unconscious meanings of the symptoms and maladaptive behavior* that the therapist and patient will actively pursue. It also opens the way for future variations or additions as they unfold. It should never become a rigid construct into which subsequent data are squeezed. *From start to finish this will be an evolving formulation subject to review and revision as the result of continued active and engaged listening.*

The formulation should be shared with the patient by the fourth to sixth session in the 24-session time-limited treatment and verbalized as a partial understanding for the scrutiny of the patient and therapist, who may tweak specifics and alter the formulation, making it a co-construction that can be held as a tentative encapsulation of the meaning of symptoms. The collaborative patient-therapist dyad can acknowledge this formulation, review it, and work on it as new experiences arise. It should include a partial understanding of the anxiety symptoms from the perspective of their emotional meanings and the protective adaptations that have been used by the patient. The formula is *dynamic* in the sense that it reflects tensions within between desire and constraint at the behest of internal conscience or a sense of danger. It also is dynamic insofar as various affective dynamisms are in flux, and change in poignancy is frequent because of gradual affective relief as understanding and greater trust take hold.

4.1.2. Common Psychodynamic Constellations

Experience with anxious children has indicated a number of recurrent constellations that often make up these formulations (Box 4.3). The following list is not exhaustive, but it contains some of the most common constellations that have been empirically collated.

BOX 4.3 Common Psychodynamic Constellations

1. Fear of passive abandonment in ambivalent relationship to attachment object (i.e., parents, caretaker): especially in agoraphobia
2. Fear of own aggressive and angry affects and fantasies leading to defensive denial, repression, and avoidance
3. Fear of exhibitionistic narcissistic (sexual and angry) wishes: especially in social phobias
4. Ambivalence regarding achievement of adult autonomy and readiness for independence: especially in adolescence
5. Disturbed by daydreams, fantasies, and dreams regarding sexual identity and direction of desire: common conflicts in adolescence
6. Fear of bodily harm leading to phobic avoidance of sports and engagement in age-related vigorous competitive encounters

They are bare-boned structures that must be fleshed out by individual experiences of our patients:

1. Fear of *separation from parents* (or other primary caretaker), who are the primary love objects, and related ambivalence concerning impending age-appropriate autonomy.
2. Difficulties experiencing/acknowledging *rage and anger/mixed aggressive and loving, i.e., ambivalent feelings* toward attachment objects, such as parents/siblings or their stand-ins. *One example:* Anxious children sometimes develop compulsive acts that seem to have no meaning, such as turning pointed objects, even shoes, in directions away from siblings to magically protect them from their own angry thoughts.
3. Conflicts concerning *growing awareness of sexual arousal* in relation to realization of sexual identity. Newly formed sexual fantasies about exposure of body, self-states, or masturbation fantasies may dominate the picture, *leading to social removal and newly experienced general caution in public displays.* This is common in social phobia and stage fright and less frequent in generalized anxiety disorder and separation anxiety disorder. Small guideposts to strongly held mixed or ambivalent feelings abound. *One example:* The preteen who wears a scanty bathing suit is frequently tugging up and down to cover budding signs of sexuality while also wishing to display her new shape anxiously.
4. *Disturbing daydreams and preconscious* (see Glossary) *fantasies* that occupy the teen at bedtime or when alone that seem to haunt consciousness, intruding on social competence. Anxiety at bedtime often relates to daily review of happenings and wishful fantasies that emerge as conscious controls lapse with approaching sleep. Such regressions are often frightening and create new arousal rather than relaxation.
5. Guilty preoccupations with a variety of *fantasied transgressions.* Anxious youngsters repetitively review possible wrong interpretations of prior conversations or go over what they said interminably, chastising themselves about what might have been said. *The anxiety thus generated may lead to obsessional/ruminative thoughts of regret* and imagined *loss,* followed by a *need for reassurance.*

4.1.3. Psychotherapeutic Techniques

The therapeutic encounter at the beginning is inquiring and exploratory, with great sensitivity to patients' weak or "shy" spots. The surface behavior and affective responses are the guideposts to understanding and cooperation. Anxious children and adolescents often tear at the therapist's heartstrings, imploring the therapist for fast fixes to feel less anxious, techniques to forestall the unpleasant feelings, and tricks to undo their sad plight. These variables have to be considered in the transference/countertransference and often dictate the sense of urgency to move to action in the general inquiry. The patient is enlisted as a coinvestigator in uncovering the roots of the discomfort and the meanings of the worries. The transference and a rapidly unfolding emotional understanding provide temporary buffers against the sense of being overwhelmed and the wish for an immediate fix. If prominent, the emergence of old behavioral patterns should be approached early and explained as repeating prior behaviors, often with parents who may have been the original target/recipient of cajoling, repetitive obsessional questioning, and regressive cuddling, which are yet other manifestations of children's anxieties. These adaptive surface behaviors reflect the patient's sense of how they get on in the world and their cover for the dangers of maturation.

During the initial inquiry, the therapist often meets with restricted exposure and shy removal and general defensiveness. These defenses should be approached early and interpreted as deterrents to the purpose of the therapy, which will be devoted to the understanding and uncovering of secrets to be discovered and thoughts that are associated with either guilt or shame. Thus the general rule of interpreting the defenses is the first order of business before the unconscious or conscious fantasies are exposed and examined. A common example of this may be seen in school reluctance, which is a maladaptation covering separation anxiety and the sense of vulnerability experienced when away from the caretaker or home in all its connotations.

Case Vignette

A 13-year-old girl protested to her mother that she was cruel to send her to school when she felt so anxious and asked if her mother would still love her if she remained at home. Her wise mother responded that love is there always, but that respect had to be earned. Therapists must enjoin all agencies of the child's inner concerns that will support their affective aims. This brief exchange suggests some routes that may undercut wrong thinking and *replace the affective worries* (being anxious about going to school and not being loved anymore by mother) *with more adaptive and autonomy-syntonic aims* (going to school despite worries, feeling proud as a result and earning respect for it).

After a formulation or interpretation is voiced in words, both observers can use it as a handle to be grasped in repetition and considered in consciousness and reflected on for future work.

General Guidelines and Examples of Psychotherapeutic Techniques for the Opening Phase

Refer to Box 4.4.

1. Sensitive *inquiry* and *exploration* into anxiety symptoms with the child/teen as "guide"
2. Awareness in the therapist of beginning *transference development* of patient toward therapist
3. Awareness in the therapist of own *countertransference reactions*, for example, if leaning toward quickly assuaging patients' distress, or rescuing rather than understanding
4. Enlist the patient as coinvestigator *to establish a collaborative working relationship*
5. Address *maladaptive behavioral patterns early* but sensitively
6. *Interpret defenses* before addressing conscious or unconscious fantasies (Box 4.5)

BOX 4.4 Dynamic Techniques

1. Listening
2. Questioning specific elements of stories/clarification
3. Clarifying
4. Confronting
5. Linkages to anxiety symptoms (past, present, transference)
6. Play and talk linkage with anxiety focus
7. Interpreting:
   Anxiety symptoms
   Internal (defense/wish)
   External interactions with others
   Transference
   Dreams/drawings

The following two vignettes of six-year-old Sally and 16-year-old Laura give examples of the opening phase of treatment with a school-aged child and a teen-aged patient.

4.1.4. Case: Six-Year-Old Sally

Sally was a six-year-old girl referred to therapy with generalized anxiety disorder who had exhibited caution at school and uneasy friendships associated with separation anxiety. This was exemplified by clinging and worrying each time her mother left her with a sitter and by dallying at dressing and breakfast before going to school, engendering her mother's impatience and chiding her because she was making everyone late, including her older sister. Such events often resulted in shouting and arguments and ultimately with Sally protesting that her mother was unfair and that Sally hated her. Reconciliations and remorse often followed, with promises to do better and requests for reassurance that her mother would be there for pick-up and not be late.

During the initial therapeutic meetings, Sally wanted her mother to join her in the consulting room. She was, however, willing to go in on her own on the contingency that if she felt uncomfortable she could touch base, refuel, and then resume. Her mother promised not to leave before she was finished. When in the room, the therapist noted that Sally seemed worried that her mother would break her promise. Sally did not say anything and seemed reluctant to talk or to even make eye contact. She was offered a stack of paper and decided to draw. She soon shared her drawings with the therapist and asked to make a book to which the therapist would add a text dictated by Sally. This became the dominant medium of exchange that lessened the defensive barriers and gave her the opportunity to further understand her unspoken fantasies. The story unfolded over the next three sessions

BOX 4.5 Defense Mechanisms

Defenses are unconscious psychological mechanisms activated by undetected (signal) anxiety in response to external or internal mental constellations that function to prevent the emergence of disorganizing or panic-level anxiety. Defenses are normal psychological functions that protect us from unacceptable ideas that conflict with cultural or personal moral constraints, they can be maladaptive if used (excessively) to resolve unconscious conflicts. See also Glossary.

Repression: The cardinal defense that maintains psychic equilibrium by not permitting unconscious fantasies into awareness

Suppression: Utilizes a *conscious* component to hide a secret wish

Reaction formation: Defends against an unconscious fantasy by enacting the opposite, for example, the "do-gooder" compliant child who covers hidden hostility at the bully, or a behaviorally passive child who covers anger and destructive rage by appearing harmless

Turning into opposite: A conscious fantasy or wish that covers an unconscious idea as in the case of reaction formation

Focus on past/focus on present: A partially conscious or unconscious choice of focus; for example, when the patient chooses to focus on either the past or the present, he/she is likely defending against the time period not mentioned, and it is likely that the omitted events and thoughts concerning that period are high in emotional valence

Identification: The incorporation of traits and features of a significant attachment figure (i.e., parent) defending against loss of that person by becoming that person in fantasy or enacting that personality trait

Projection: The process of transferring onto another person the wishes and traits that are not acknowledged or owned in oneself (e.g., angry/aggressive feelings)

Denial: A reality-distorting defense designed to avoid a perception that is disturbing

Displacement: Transferring the object of anxiety to a benign person, place, or thing as a means of avoiding recognition of an anxiety-generating experience that would feel dangerous to the child's sense of integrity

Somatization: A defense that permits recognition of bodily disturbance while omitting conscious recognition of anxiety; for example, the bodily focus is often determined by a diathesis or former focus of a physical disorder and leads to secondary gain (e.g., attention to the body, medical attention) and displacement from conscious conflict

accompanied by sketchy drawings. The story had some kinship to the culturally available "Red Riding Hood" and was a derivative tale of going off into unknown quarters seeking her lost grandmother. The streets were full of dangers that the little girl evaded only to arrive at granny's to find a large dangerous-looking dog that blocked entry. The fictional heroine was paralyzed and could not decide whether to run or defy the danger. Suddenly the scene changed, and she was safe in her grandmother's lap sitting by a fire, all warm and happy.

Therapist's Understanding of the Sessions With Sally

The therapist extracted the theme of separation anxiety and wish for bravery (exposing self to dangers and evading them) from the story. He connected these themes to Sally's relationship with her mother and noted her fear that her mother might not like her to be on her own and that she, Sally, was fearful that her mother was angry. Her mother's angry displays during Sally's tantrums, represented in the story by the dangerous-looking dog, frightened Sally so that in the end she felt the urgent need to return and become a little girl safe in grandmother's lap. In the initial formulation, the substitution of a receptive grandmother for her mother was left to be understood as time progressed.

The link to a recent discovery became a further concrete advance about her own history. The therapist and Sally learned that Sally had been adopted. This revelation permitted the mental exploration for a loving other parent, personified in the story by grandma. This identity was made explicit by the therapist. At the same time, wishes to have another, better mother had to be defended against fear that her adoptive mother would not like an intruder to come between her and the patient. Her story drawing and telling thus became the shadow narrative of her fantasies of family romance that superseded her adoptive family *that had to be disguised in order to protect her core relationship to her mother,* as well as *to protect her from the terrible guilt that such fantasies, if openly acknowledged, would engender anger and rejection. Sally also struggled, as many adopted children do, with the idea that she had been rejected by her birth mother, threatening her adoptive parental relationships with heightened fear of rejection.*

This initial formulation then became the posited dynamism of her struggle and was revisited many times during the remainder of the therapy in many new and creative formats. The various forms were reinterpreted, and the many variant stories were shown to be versions of the same worries until the child began to be able to grasp the singular meaning of her anxiety and apply conscious means to master the fears.

4.1.5. Case: Sixteen-Year-Old Laura

Laura, who we have already met in Chapter 3, was age 16 when she came to treatment unable to sleep in her own bed and anxious that her mother had been run down in the street or was mugged when her mother was a bit late for dinner. Laura had recurrent obsessional thoughts that she needed to call her mother, although she had been admonished not to interrupt her at work during the day. Laura was reluctant to join her friends on weekends at parties and usually chose instead to visit her grandmother with her little brother at the beach. She was diagnosed with general anxiety disorder and separation anxiety disorder.

The initial meetings were spent with Laura telling the therapist about how her father had died four years earlier and that she had been woken by her mother to help in the middle of the night before the ambulance carried him in a near-death state to the hospital. The mother went through a complicated mourning process for a year. She could not sustain her job, and the family was soon close to destitute. When the mother found work, she was erratic in her attendance because she suffered from a low-grade chronic physical illness. Laura had adored her father and had been in the throes of a prepubertal battle with her mother when he died.

Beginning Phase of Treatment

Laura easily acknowledged having violent and angry thoughts directed at her mother, only to become frightened that her mother too might die and leave her alone. She worried about getting angry or expressing anger at her mother, and her secret wish was to be grown up enough to retaliate and go off to college and leave her mother alone. In contrast to this fantasy of independence, Laura slept in her mother's bed for fear her mother might die in the night, as had her father. The core focus of her anxiety was gradually formulated in terms of *her fear that her anger could kill* and that *her mother would discover that Laura wanted her death* so that, in fantasy, she could carry on living with the protection of her father. This fantasy was regressive and impossible, of course, because Laura was acutely aware that her father had died, which she experienced as abandonment.

Once more these core fantasies became the meaningful theme of many variant symptoms and obsessions that emerged at a later phase of the treatment.

4.1.6. Opening Phase: Thirteen-Year-Old Tom

We met Tom, a 13-year-old seventh-grader, in Chapter 1. We will now hear how his treatment unfolded. His *Diagnostic and Statistical Manual of Mental Disorders, fourth edition* (DSM-IV) (3) diagnoses at evaluation on the Anxiety Disorders Interview Schedule, Child and Parent Version (ADIS-C/P) (4) were: social phobia 6/8, separation anxiety disorder 5/8, and dysthymic disorder 4/8. He was also diagnosed with a mild nonverbal learning disability. Separation anxiety was complicated by the fact that Tom's mother had become a "phobic companion" and arranged situations for Tom in ways such that he did not experience his separation anxiety. For example, she avoided ever leaving him alone or with a sitter. This contributed to Tom not scoring higher for separation anxiety disorder on the ADIS.

The first phase of treatment resulted in the following psychodynamic formulation:

Tom's chronic symptoms had become more prominent and ego dystonic as he became a young teen and began to feel the pull of individuation. Being anxious, shy, and scared now interfered more with his life and was increasingly developmentally incongruous. His attachment to his mother prevented him from more independent age-appropriate activities with peers. His fears of separation also hid his angry emotions, which had aggressive, as well as assertive, aspects. One aspect of his angry feelings was that the excessive closeness with his mother (a not uncommon dynamism) made him feel small and infantile. He wished to be a maturing and more independent young man and strong like father one day. While these were things he wanted for himself, they were frightening at the same time because they were incompatible with being a dependent and at all times cared-for young child. His social shyness was also an expression of conflict, and his desire to be the center of attention and to be in control of things was expressed in his assertive love of performing magic tricks and being admired as he controlled his audience.

Clinical Encounters

Tom presented as a handsome young teen, looking somewhat younger than his age. He easily engaged, was verbal, and had a fine sense of humor. Contrasting with his somewhat younger appearance, he at times sounded precocious and "wiser" than one might expect of a boy his age, reflecting the predominantly adult company he was in, except for the hours he spent in school.

For the first few visits he was dropped off by a family member.

Tom's style of engaging with the therapist was that he would begin to "chat" about his day or the previous weekend. It was rare that he directly addressed his worries or even presented them as his reason for being in the therapist's office. He *avoided* the topic of his anxieties, and they seemed at first to be largely ego syntonic.

Listening to Tom's narrative of his daily life, the therapist paid careful attention to identify themes that related to his anxieties and helped Tom to *elaborate* on his fears. For example, Tom mentioned that he called his mother a lot during the day. The therapist asked Tom to say more about this, which led to Tom elaborating: he wanted to make sure that his mother was alright (note that his mother is healthy), but as he thought more about this, he began to realize and could therefore express verbally that *he was the one who worried about being away from his mother*. This elaboration helped Tom reflect on his own mind, and he realized that calling his mother frequently was not about her but instead was about him in relation to her. This is an example of a beginning improvement in Tom's reflective functioning.

Another such instance was when Tom related that he did not have difficulties socializing in general but that he found it stressful to meet new kids. Again, using the technique of *elaboration*, the therapist asked Tom to say more about such situations. Tom then described that he was worried kids would not acknowledge him or would make fun of him if he gave a wrong answer in class. This led to the therapist asking what his experience with such situations had been, only to learn that Tom never had such an experience in real life but that he *imagined* it. Thus the therapist helped Tom identify that there was a *magical quality* to this fear, which led to maladaptive, avoidant behavior. This, in turn, interfered with age-appropriate behavior, such as socializing with peers, as well as engaging fully academically.

When Tom talked about an experience that showed that his magical fears did not correspond to reality, the therapist pointed it out and *addressed the maladaptive defense*: Tom went to a new place, and another child said "hi" back after he said "hi." The therapist pointed out that this was just what he was afraid of, the child not saying "hi," but that it did not happen that way. In a similar vein, when Tom related that he says, "I don't know" when called on in class because of his fear of giving a wrong response, the therapist pointed out to Tom: "You are so worried about giving an incorrect response that not knowing seems better than the risk of giving a wrong response," again pointing out a *maladaptive defensive pattern. The focus on defense rather than the content of the fear enables a more open and safe arena in which he could approach his more guarded inner experiences and unconscious fantasies.* When Tom got an inspiration for an essay from an object in the therapist's office and said to the therapist: "You gave me the idea," the therapist clarified that it was Tom who had the idea but that he got it while with the therapist. With this intervention, the therapist *clarified a distortion* that Tom frequently employed, imagining himself less an agent than he was. The therapist thereby emphasized Tom's *agency and autonomy*.

When Tom, for the first time began to come alone to his appointment (which was age-appropriate behavior, considering the circumstances), the therapist made this explicit and used it to address Tom's anxieties: the therapist said to Tom, "We have understood together that doing things alone, without your mom, worried you a lot, but now you are starting to try it yourself. What was it to like to come over alone?" Tom articulated that he felt quite safe because he came from his friend who lives close by. However, he continued, it was still a big and scary step for him that reminded him of the attack by older youth not long ago.

Another defensive pattern the therapist noted was his habit of making bad or not so good things look better than they really were, often finding good or funny aspects *(reversal of affect and exaggerated use of humor)*. A moderate use of this type of defense can be adaptive. In Tom's case, however, it served the *avoidance of negative affects such as sadness and disappointment.* One of many examples ("redundancy of themes," see also the discussion of the CAPP middle phase) was when Tom's plans to go to a long-awaited movie premier with his friend fell through because his friend was sick. He was only able to express minimal disappointment and shifted quickly ("affective shift," see also the discussion of the CAPP middle phase) to identifying positive aspects of the cancellation, notably emphasizing that he used the free time to study for a test. The therapist and Tom developed their own language for this phenomenon and called it Tom looking at the "sunny side of things," noting that this seemed much easier for him than to experience sadness or disappointment.

Tom's attraction to magic and demonstrating his tricks in front of an audience stood in contrast to his social shyness and expressed Tom's *conflicted wish to be the center of attention*. The therapist chose to address this to help Tom begin to see how his social avoidance was contrasted by his enjoyment in social display. The hope would be that at some point in the future Tom could acknowledge how much he wanted to be seen and have an audience and that his social avoidance protected him against the acceptance of this desire, which he experienced as shameful. Such interpretations are delicate and have to be done with particular caution and tact to avoid the patient feeling exposed or criticized. In this instance, the therapist decided to only point out to Tom that he enjoyed showing how skilled he was at magic tricks and that he liked to be the only one who knows about secrets. This technique is a *defense interpretation.*

The therapist noted during the opening phase of treatment that Tom employed *counterphobic defenses.* He talked excitedly and with visible pleasure about scary-sounding storms, ambulances, fallen trees, and car accidents that he had heard of but that did not directly affect him. Counterphobic defenses are a psychological strategy not only to feel in control of one's anxiety but also to feel the opposite emotion, in this case being courageous and "tough." The therapist thought that Tom might not yet be able to relate to an interpretation of this defense and waited until the next phase of treatment.

As the treatment moved toward the end of the opening phase, Tom expressed his increasing attachment to the therapist, mainly by commenting repeatedly that he liked the appearance of the therapist's consulting room. The therapist was acutely aware of the need to address the time-limited nature of treatment, although it was still relatively early in treatment. The therapist commented to Tom that it might be hard to finish a few months from now because he so much liked coming now (*transference-focused comment*).

Summary of Psychotherapeutic Techniques Used During the Opening Phase of Tom's Treatment

Refer to Box 4.4.

1. Encourage the patient to elaborate specifically and in detail his anxiety-related thoughts, worries, fantasies, and anxiety triggers.
2. Identify and begin to address defenses, such as magical thinking, counterphobic behaviors, and reversal of affect.
3. Demonstrate to the patient that the symptoms have emotionally connected meaning, with the goal of improvement of symptom-specific reflective functioning.

4.2. CAPP Middle Phase

The middle phase of this psychodynamic psychotherapy follows the initial plan of listening carefully to the patient's words and inflections as he/she tells his/her story, the quotidian events of life, with a specific focus on the troubling incidents that arouse anxiety. In this mode of permission to choose the topic, the most trivial story may become disturbing and emotionally salient. *The narratives now feel familiar and seemingly repetitious or redundant, both in theme and content*, although new narratives also commonly arise. The therapist must permit the patient to tell his/her individual experiences in his/her own personal style and manner. While the therapist is attentive to the immediate needs of the patient, his/her interventions carry the patient back to the earlier formulation by registering similarities in the current play or narrative to themes already discussed by both participants. New stories may lead to exposing other themes that plague the child in addition to the primary dynamism. Among the five most common dynamisms outlined earlier, there may be a shift in primacy of concern. The therapist joins the dialogue and encourages reflection and continuing curiosity regarding the meaning of the child's experience. It is all too easy to falter in what seems to be a randomness of the presentation. This seeming randomness may serve a defensive function, "protecting" the child from the underlying troublesome emotions and thoughts. The therapist must also keep in mind that current concerns at the center of the presentation (rather than the anxiety symptoms) have priority for the patient and should be acknowledged. It would be counterproductive to become too diligent in only focusing on the central task of the therapy and not also meeting the child in the "here and now."

As the therapist begins to see patterns of expression and storyline in addition to attempts to consciously or unconsciously bring the therapist into the dialogue, the very complaints regarding friends and family invariably seem all too present in experiences within the treatment or in transparently displaced complaints about the relationship with the therapist. "Transferences" (a re-experiencing of familiar, early life relationship patterns, now with the therapist) are noted and articulated so that the *patient can begin to understand his/her patterns as they intrude into this new relationship*. When feelings about the therapist are negative, they may begin to interfere with the therapeutic process, and they therefore must be verbalized and introduced into the dialogue. However, premature leaps to a focus on the transference can be tricky. If focused on too early and not supported by the affective valence of immediate concerns, they can seem just plain wrong, intellectualized, and even glib.

To tell a child that what he/she is saying or doing suggests, for example, that the patient is angry with the therapist or frightened of being abandoned by therapist carries no weight compared with the patient's long commitment that a parent is the center of his/her worries.

A cooperative inquiry into the directedness of the affect, sudden withdrawal, or relative muteness in session, all of which have their internal reasons, creates a better climate for a transference interpretation because it grows out of the common experience between therapist and child that can be cited.

As the therapist listens for themes that underlie anxiety symptoms, the therapist focuses specifically and selectively on the following *middle phase phenomena* (examples follow the list):

1. Redundancies. Themes being repeated or re-enacted in different places, ways, or relationships and settings, including in the transference. Triggers for anxiety are

often repeated in stories, as are specific interpersonal constellations. The emotional arousal may be redundant, as may the defenses that are called into play during certain encounters.

2. Seeking a homology of narratives that emerge in diverse communications, whether through play or talk. The form of the stories or play often follows patterns that are not recognized by the patient until attention is drawn to them in the clinical encounter.

3. Changes in either vehicle or medium of expression (change from play to talk, or from one play/talk theme to another play/talk theme) as well as affective shifts (e.g., suddenly sad to giddy) are remarked on by the therapist to the child in their function as defense, confession, or both. Some refer to such shifts and changes as surface behavior in response to the child's inner cognitions and emotional arousal.

During this phase, the patient makes progress by actively tracking his/her anxiety and drilling to deeper understandings. There will be many episodes concerning mastery of former regressive tendencies and attempts to enter better adaptive stances that help in life. If changes are sudden and not accompanied by a more gradual understanding, the therapist must keep in mind that they may be *counterphobic enactments*, unconsciously designed to please the therapist or parents or to minimize the impact of the anxiety to oneself. Counterphobia refers to a psychological mechanism in which rather than avoiding anxiety-inducing situations, the individual actively seeks them out in an attempt to master or control the feared situation and deny the gravity of anxiety. Many youngsters believe that if they do what the grown-ups wish, it will gain approval. *However, such behavior does not serve to alter anxiety.* Such behaviors, which can represent transference enactments and can reflect a wish to please a therapist by appearing "better," should ultimately be tactfully exposed and hopefully replaced with behaviors that represent attempts toward maturation that rest on growing resolution of inner conflicts and a clearer relationship to reality.

Moves toward health should be acknowledged and explored so that mentalizing work can be placed on better conscious scaffolding that can be revisited by the patient. Such *improvements in reflective functioning* allow the symptoms to begin to be considered as unnatural, or ego alien, and neither as a default mechanism nor a focus for catastrophe. These newly formulated products of understanding are cast in a verbal form that can be remembered and reconsidered as a signal to guard against former poor adaptation.

The possibility of encouraging self-conscious reappraisal and reflection on new events as being similar to earlier experiences is the essence of improvement in reflective functioning. The therapist's goal is to replace what seem to be automatic maladaptive behaviors and thoughts with new adaptive behaviors and a wider range of possible responses. During CAPP, as the process progresses, the now more reflective child can inwardly say, "This situation is like the one I talked about with my therapist, and I do not have to be afraid or continue to act as I did last week." Such reflection soon broadens the scope of possible responses and breaks the rigidity of the former set encounters.

4.2.1. Case: Seven-Year-Old Max

Max is a seven-year-old boy who was referred because of a recent tendency toward selective mutism and increasing anxiety following an episode of bullying. He had an earlier history of shyness and clinging behavior that warranted a diagnosis of separation anxiety disorder.

Clinical Encounter

Max was relatively nonverbal and began each session by going to the cars. He repeatedly enacted a scene in which a law-abiding car, just moving along slowly and stopping at signs, is sideswiped by a more aggressively moving car. However, at each accident a vigilant police car was there to apprehend the offender and call emergency medical services, who rescue the driver.

Max has told the therapist that he fears going to school because he doesn't want to be teased by a bully and that he fears his mother will not be there to pick him up at day's end.

During an iteration of the repetitive play, the therapist mentioned that the "guy in the car is lucky to have a very careful and watching police man."

> MAX: Yeah.
> THERAPIST: But you worry your mother is not so careful and not going to be there to pick you up.
> MAX: But she's been there lately.
> THERAPIST: That's great and I know you'd like to be sure, but in the beginning, you weren't so sure, so in your game you always have the cops there.

This brief play/talk sequence offers an example of all three repetitive forms:

1. *Repeated themes in play:* Max plays out the same scene over and over again.
2. *Homology in verbal and play media or representation:* Max expresses the same content in his play and with his words.
3. *Defenses are revealed in the translation from play to talk:* Max demonstrated in his play the constellation of a careful driver being threatened by a "bully" driver, and a cop helping out. When translated into words with the help of the therapist, the events in his life could be made more understandable to him and replayed parsimoniously and reconsidered over time.

4.2.2. Case: Eight-Year-Old Paula

Paula, an eight-year-old girl in second grade, with separation anxiety disorder since preschool and social phobia, was having severe difficulties at school with several girls, all of whom made fun of her. Paula, who was always extremely shy, had retreated to near-silence. Her mother reported that the teacher told her that Paula mostly answered questions in school in a monosyllabic whisper and that she sat alone at recess. Paula told her mother that she was frightened to speak up because the other girls just made fun of her or talked over her. She repeatedly mentioned to the therapist that she could never think of "what to say."

Clinical Encounter

The following vignette comes from the middle of an exuberant session in which Paula had been playing the game "house guest," which she had invented during her therapy.

In this game, Glinda, a glamorous older girl doll, comes to visit the doll Sally's family as a houseguest for an extended visit. Sally becomes so excited about the glamorous girl's visit that she follows her everywhere and constantly bothers her. The older girl is nice and sweet to Sally, but Paula is clear in acting this part that she and Glinda think Sally's slavish, excited attention to the older girl is embarrassing.

PAULA (AS THE MOTHER DOLL): Sally, give Glinda a little space, she just arrived, please don't go through her bags, she wants to get settled in.
PAULA (AS GLINDA): Oh, no, Mrs. P, it's fine, Sally's just little. (Paula makes a face— Glinda is just tolerating Sally enough to be nice.)
PAULA (AS SALLY): I want to play with you all the time, Glinda! I want to share a bedroom with you! I want to take you to school with me!

Suddenly, Paula's tone changed, and she looked downcast.

PAULA (AS HERSELF): I'm sick of this game, let's do something else.
THERAPIST: It looks as though something suddenly bothered you about this game.
PAULA: Not really.
THERAPIST: I was a little bit wondering about whether it might have been when Sally started talking about school.
PAULA: I don't know.

Therapist's Understanding of the Sequence

The representative play demonstrates the *repetitive themes* of idealization, slavish devotion to others, and the anxiety that accrues in realization of lessened self-esteem leading to withdrawal. Within the therapy, the therapist noticed the *change in vehicle of expression from play to talk in the context of a mood change*. This provided a chance to help the patient to recognize the signal, school, that linked play to life with anxiety.

4.2.3. Case: Ten-Year-Old Matt

Matt, 10-years old, was referred to treatment for generalized anxiety disorder just as he was approaching new opportunities to show his growing capacities to tolerate his anxiety. He grasped onto the hope that his therapist would carry him through into puberty and a more mature stance at school. Matt told of an incident during the middle phase of his treatment that represents an attempt to master his reluctance and anxiety:

Clinical Encounter

THERAPIST: How did all this begin?

MATT: I don't know, it just started 4 weeks ago.

THERAPIST: That's pretty specific!

MATT: Yeah.

THERAPIST: Yeah what?

MATT: I was walking home from school.

THERAPIST: You go home alone?

MATT: I only live around the corner and my mom said it was ok to try, my friend Ira does it too.

THERAPIST: You usually go with him?

MATT: Not that day.

THERAPIST: It must have been hard to be all alone.

MATT: I didn't know he was sick when I went to school.

THERAPIST: So you were trying something new that day.

MATT: I'm already 10 years old.

THERAPIST: So you think you should have been able to do it.

MATT: I was doing it and then my heart started beating, and I thought I saw this tough bully at the corner, and I panicked.

THERAPIST: You thought you saw him?

MATT: Yeah, but it was my imagination.

THERAPIST: Were you thinking something else before you had the scary feeling?

MATT: Yeah, I wished Ira was there, or that my mother would be there.

THERAPIST: So your feeling came after you thought you were alone and that you were in danger.

MATT: That bully is real danger.

THERAPIST: But you only thought he was there.

MATT: I know—I was scared to go home alone.

Therapist's Understanding of the Sequence

Matt, who uses language as his primary medium to communicate with the therapist, constructs his narrative and reveals his anxiety using the *defensive cover that the worry was a realistic fear*, requiring the therapist to remind the patient that *the imagined bully emerged in consciousness as he realized that he lacked a buffering companion who stood for his mother*.

The examples of Max, Paula, and Matt exemplify techniques used in the middle phase of treatment. They provide a framework for *repetitive therapeutic actions* concerning linkages within and among the themes, between the play/talk and current realities at home, school, and the past, and, when possible, in the transference.

4.2.4. Linkages Between Themes

The therapist actively makes linkages between:

1. Behaviors in the session, such as the child's narratives, which reveal *similar ways or recurrent themes* in which the child sees himself/herself in different relationships or settings
2. The *transference,* that is, the child's emotional experience in relation to the therapist that can be easily referenced in terms of *similarities in other relationships* that are meaningful
3. The themes that are cast in talk or play and their relationship to the child's past experiences. Linkages between form of a story or demonstrated human interactions derived from past and present comprise opportunities to condense and integrate disparate information that can be expressed verbally. Sometimes information obtained from the parents can be helpful in formulations.

All of these interventions help the patient to elaborate on fantasies preceding or during the anxious events. In Matt's case, for example, the exploration of the context of symptom onset helped the elaboration of his fantasy that the bully was actually physically present.

4.2.5. Interpretations

The therapist makes interpretations by explaining behavior and fears in context:

1. In the process of the play during session, and in the themes (content) revealed by the play
2. Focusing on the defenses, either what is making it difficult to play/talk or the defensive significance of the anxiety, for example, a child preventing parental fighting by always being with mother—hence serving as a "guard"
3. Themes in play, significance of underlying fantasies—particularly as they concern anxiety
4. Transference, which becomes more important toward termination of therapy when the therapist actively reminds the child that therapy is ending and the child perforce has to focus on the relationship with the therapist ending

The following examples of talking and playing children demonstrate the complex interplay of *denial of anxiety* and *admission of feelings of inadequacy and weakness,* and the *wish for a sense of power and conviction about control of bad feelings.* Open displays or protests that can resemble bravado may conceal a sense of inadequate abilities to navigate the life tasks that are related to developmental stage. While these dynamics may appear at any stage of the therapy, it is wise to interpret them during the middle phase when the therapeutic alliance is strong and unclouded by looming termination.

4.2.6. Case: Ten-Year-Old Jim

Jim at 10 years old suffers from generalized anxiety disorder but also is a child with narcissistic traits whose reality was shattered by not always succeeding. He tried to cover his failings with a brave front. The following segment elaborates a failed attempt to be more mature and a therapeutic intervention that offers some internal tolerance for a sense of vulnerability.

Clinical Encounter

Jim tells repeatedly of his prowess at video games and in checkers with his little brother but avoids the fact that he cries easily and cowers when anyone raises their voice. He describes his teacher as a witch—the therapist suggests that though he does OK in class, a witch is a scary idea.

JIM: Yeah, but I've got her number.

THERAPIST: So now you are not scared because you are tougher?

JIM: I'm not a wimp.

THERAPIST: I can see that; but even tough people sometimes feel scared.

JIM: My dad says I'm like him.

THERAPIST: I'm sure that makes you proud.

JIM: Yeah, but you know my mom keeps yelling at him, and he doesn't answer.

THERAPIST: That makes you think what?

JIM: Maybe being like him in everything isn't so good.

THERAPIST: So even strong people can have times when they are scared.

JIM: I guess so, you know, even my little brother is beginning to worry me, he might beat me at the game we play sooner than I expected.

THERAPIST: You know, maybe he will get better as he gets older and you too will be strong and win a lot of the time when you are bigger, but right now it's OK to feel weaker sometimes and not have to be the best all the time. I sometimes think that you talk so tough a lot to try to tell yourself that you aren't worried and because you feel you're smaller than you want to be.

Therapist's Understanding of the Sequence

The therapist's remark is supportive and interpretative at the same time. He makes it acceptable for Jim to feel vulnerable and does not criticize him for his bravado but offers his understanding of it: Jim "talks tough" to feel better, rather than acknowledging that he feels small and threatened.

4.2.7. Case: Nine-Year-Old Lilly

Lilly, a nervous nine-year-old adopted girl, worried about almost everything, usually involving her grades in school. She was an excellent student but fretted about each test, demanding of herself that she get 100. She also worried about her social standing at her upper-class girls' school, her athletic performance, and, secretly, whether she looked too different from her parents and hence whether anyone would be able to "tell" that she was adopted. Despite her general shyness, Lilly had developed a habit of vociferously arguing with teachers in school, to the point that her parents had been summoned to school. She was diagnosed with generalized anxiety disorder.

Clinical Encounter

Although going to therapy was a "deep six" secret, she very much enjoyed coming and having "my own special doctor" to whom she could tell "everything." "Now this is deep, and dark, and secret," she occasionally said.

Lilly had a habit of throwing many things around the office as she played and talked: packs of cards, crayons, packs of paper, trucks. "It looks like a bomb hit the place," she would sigh with satisfaction toward the end of the session.

> THERAPIST: You seem really pleased to have made such a mess. I can't help wondering why you always do this.
> LILLY (GRINNING): I have no idea!
> THERAPIST: If I didn't know better, I would really think you like doing this.
> LILLY (GRINS): You think so? . . . Are you mad at me? (smiling broadly).

One day, during the extended cleanup, which had become a routine in which Lilly was a somewhat reluctant participant:

> THERAPIST: You know, I'm pretty struck by your asking if I'm mad at you. Do you think you might be trying to get me mad with all of this mess all the time?
> LILLY (GRINNING): I dunno.
> THERAPIST: I sometimes think that you may try to make me mad here, just like you do with some of the teachers at school. I think you want to see if they'll get so mad that they throw you out.
> LILLY (SERIOUS SUDDENLY): Maybe.

Therapist's Understanding of the Session With Lilly

This latter example brings us to a more complex repetitive behavior that seems contrary to what the child openly wishes to be aiming for. It involves turning *passive dependency into pseudo-assertiveness,* an activity akin to a "you can't fire me, I quit!" dynamic. In this scenario, a nontherapist partner to the behavior, like a teacher in school, might be tempted to respond to the set-up derived from the patient's fantasy by acting in the predicted expected manner, such as reprimanding the child. As shown in Lilly's case, the therapist's understanding of her unruly behavior and the subsequent interpretation that Lilly might provoke being kicked out, which could constitute a maladaptive way to take control of the past traumatic experience of being giving up for adoption (the latter part was not interpreted to the patient during this phase, but was later), allows Lilly and the therapist to think together about this dynamic.

4.2.8. Middle Phase: Thirteen-Year-Old Tom
Overview

The initial psychodynamic formulation that Tom's long-standing social phobia, dysthymia, and separation anxiety, to which his mother had become a phobic companion by rearranging situations so as to avoid aggravating Tom's separation anxiety, had become more troublesome to him as he was getting older and his desire for individuation had grown stronger, was confirmed and expanded.

Tom's difficulties separating from his mother started to improve. He ventured out, less separation anxious and less socially avoidant, and his mother was able to tolerate this. Parental support for growing autonomy is not to be taken for granted because some parents of separation anxious children are themselves quite separation anxious and find it difficult to tolerate their child's newfound independence. They may create, not always consciously, interferences with the treatment progress. This was not the case with Tom and his family.

As treatment progressed, Tom became more aware of his inner life and developed a more realistic appreciation of himself.

It became clearer during this phase of treatment that Tom identified with his father and wished, timidly, albeit deeply, to be strong and manly like his father. His ambivalence toward his mother, who at times interfered with his "man-to-man" time with his father, of which he could barely get enough, was palpable but difficult for Tom to acknowledge and articulate.

Tom became increasingly attached to the therapist. This reflected a positive therapeutic alliance and translated to Tom being engaged and increasingly open in his treatment, but it simultaneously alerted the therapist to the importance of addressing the time-limited nature of the treatment early on because it was predictable that his separation anxiety was likely to re-emerge as termination approached. This would provide an important opportunity for discussion and deeper understanding.

The main defenses observed and interpreted were Tom's avoidance of negative affects by turning them into the opposite (reversal of affect), his counterphobic defenses (being excited about dangerous situations he was not directly involved in), and his magical thinking.

Examples with material from sessions will follow to illustrate how these themes presented in therapy and how the therapist addressed them with Tom.

Tom Became More Able to Acknowledge and Accept His Own Feelings

Tom and his parents decided that he should change to a less challenging school. While he had so far only emphasized that he was glad to transfer, criticizing his current school, he now said that he felt he was "bailing out." This change in narrative reflected that Tom had become more able to tolerate his own negative feelings, which resulted in increased honesty with himself and greater openness with the therapist. The therapist also acknowledged this sobering insight of Tom's by nodding in an understanding and empathic way but felt it was important to not dissuade Tom from experiencing those painful feelings or counsel or reassure him regarding his choice of school, specifically in light of the fact that he had a tendency to distance himself from painful emotions. The therapist used this moment to be emotionally available to Tom as he was experiencing a painful but not devastating feeling, from which he was likely able to move on.

Tom Ventures Out

Tom ventured out more because he was experiencing improved mood, less separation anxiety, and less social avoidance. He was making friends more easily but still had social anxiety in new settings. He successfully delivered a speech at school, something he could not have done in the past. When he proudly reported this to the therapist, she said that indeed this was wonderful and labeled his affect by saying that this achievement seemed to make him proud of himself, which he easily acknowledged.

Another instance was when one day Tom reported a "dare": he ran a small errand before the session, despite the fact that he had only five minutes to do so and risked being late, which he was not. The therapist phrased this as Tom trying out something new, taking a "calculated risk," which he was not able to allow himself previously. Tom was visibly pleased with himself. He also showed that he was more certain that his therapist would not disapprove but rather would be accepting in view of the positive meaning of this "risk adventure."

Continuing Problems: Tom Continues to Often Look at the "Sunny Side of Things"

The therapist continued to show Tom that it was often hard for him to acknowledge feelings of sadness and disappointment. Tom went on a much-anticipated trip, which was marked by multiple disappointments, but looked at the "sunny side of things," as therapist and Tom had taken to calling his tendency to make the best of things. He recounted his misadventures, including travel companions getting sick, tasteless food being served at restaurants, and being rained out in comedic ways. This was partially an *adaptive defense*, in particular because Tom used humor—he was funny and good at getting other people to laugh with him about his misadventures. However, the underlying dynamic was that he needed to *avoid feelings such as disappointment, upset, and sadness*, emotions still too painful for him to acknowledge, and that made him feel small. The therapist addressed this also in the *transference* and pointed out that Tom mostly brought up good things with the therapist and tended to stay away from his worries.

Anxious Tom Likes Scary Things: Counterphobic Defenses

The therapist noted that Tom talked with excitement about scary-sounding scenarios that he was not directly involved in. He talked about car crashes, storms, and ambulance sirens in thrilling ways. The therapist pointed out to him that it seemed interesting that he worried about things like school, what other kids thought of him, and being away from Mom, but that there were many things other people would be scared of that he found exciting! When the therapist first mentioned this, Tom acknowledged it with some measure of intrigue but did not have much to say. We will see later that he became able to work with this idea and spontaneously brought up that it was interesting that he, who was afraid of the dark, liked scary movies that had the dark as their main topic.

Tom Likes the Therapist and the Therapist's Office: Will He Become Separation Anxious at Termination?

The following exchange is an example of how a seemingly small comment Tom made was attended to by the therapist and became an opening to talking about their relationship.

One day, Tom opened the session by saying, "I have not seen you in a while," to which the therapist responded that this session took place a day later than it usually did and that this seemed to matter to Tom, reflected in his seemingly casual comment. Later during the same session, Tom revealed to the therapist for the first time how one of his magic tricks worked and added that the therapist was not likely to meet his friends and tell them the secret. The therapist interpreted that Tom could talk in session about private matters and was not worried that the therapist would reveal his secrets.

Tom then continued, expressing curiosity as to whether the therapist lived in the building the office was located. A transference-focused inquiry led to Tom talking about a fantasy related to the therapist. He imagined whether he would ever see the therapist walking down the street, which led to the therapist wondering out loud to Tom whether he ever imagined he would see the therapist after treatment had ended. After the therapist introduced the topic of termination, Tom revealed that he and his mother had talked about whether he could extend the treatment because it was so helpful to him and also to his mother because he had become more independent, which she enjoyed, too. Tom then went on, imagining knowing where the therapist lived and visiting the therapist. As Tom and the therapist discussed how much he would like that although it would not be possible, he abruptly switched topics and gaily talked about having a goodbye party at the end of treatment. This was a noticeable affective shift. When the therapist interpreted his defense and said that he was more comfortable thinking of the "sunny side of things," a party rather than sad and longing feelings, Tom suddenly said that this was exactly what his mother did routinely and that he "got it from her." This was an important insight and acknowledgement for Tom, realizing that he identified with his mother's discomfort with sadness. This was a *transference-focused intervention* as well as *fostering and enhancing of self-reflective functioning*.

4.3. CAPP Termination Phase

Although the treatment is seamless in fact and principle, it is necessary in this time-limited intervention to remind the patient that this relatively new relationship, with its frequent meetings and circumscribed intensity, will come to a close and that separation must be anticipated in fact and words so that psychological work concerning termination can be considered in the dialogue with the therapist. We recommend that at least the final eight (one-third of the entire duration of the treatment) sessions of therapy involve working on termination. There are some children who may act as if the treatment meetings can be sustained forever. Such "clingy and hungry for contact" transferences frequently occur in children who are parent-deprived and long for personal attention such as that provided in the therapy. An extreme example of such affect hunger is apparent in children with attachment disorders because of early deprivation and neglect. The other variant in such experiences is the withdrawn and emotionally blunted child whose response to early neglect is to communicate and sometimes actually feel he/she does not need anyone, as a defensive way of sustaining autonomy, but whose prospects of intimacy remain problematic. Similar responses can occur in children whose personal experiences may make them very separation anxious, or in those who cannot tolerate everyday experiences of temporary interpersonal loss.

In contrast, the brittle pseudo-autonomous and attachment-phobic child requires specific personal work directed toward facing the denial of the importance of the attachment and dependence that forces the child to play out the aloof, "I do not need you" stance that denies passivity and instead to feel completely autonomous, in an effort to disavow affective distress and separation anxiety that will inevitably emerge at termination. Some children become frankly angry and protest the treatment's ending, while others regress and re-enact the symptoms, bound as they are in dysregulated attachments, which led the child to the treatment initially. Because this is a treatment that attends to the dynamics of anxiety in the developing child, this phase is particularly salient and *subject to the coping mechanisms that are a part of the child's developmental stage and offers a proving ground for newly achieved coping skills that have been born of reflection and mastery in therapy.*

The therapist in each of these instances must attend to each child's specific capacities to cope and to the child's weak spots that led to treatment in the first place. At the same time, the therapist's own rescue fantasies have to be set aside, and the reality of a short, time-limited relationship must be introduced into the dialogue early in treatment. This may require periodic reinforcement unless the tendencies to distort the relationship as the patient's idealized new parent or new best friend can be openly discussed. It is a balance that must be struck between encouraging frankness and at the same time openly recognizing that the therapeutic relationship is "not forever." The balance, during the therapy, can be sustained by the anchoring reality, by the rising opportunities to demonstrate the patient's newly developed autonomy and competence with peers and at home, and by the opportunity to improve reflective functioning, which can be sustaining in being able to think one's way between fantasy and reality.

The focus during this period is on working in the transference as much as needed, with the therapist as a *stand-in for the depended-on object* and the need for separation. The increasing experience of newfound competence and sense of mastery that has been demonstrated during the treatment should be reviewed and emphasized. However, the stress of termination can lead to *regressive thinking* and can revive infantile feelings of needing protection, which must be acknowledged by the therapist. Prior examples drawn from the treatment that the worry and anticipation belong to fantasies of a younger, inept child-self can be helpful. The work in therapy has allowed that child to become a more confident, competent, and more age-normative youngster, who can now face a termination in this relationship and move ahead to others who are not the professionals in his life but instead are his friends and family.

Adolescents, in general, would rather often deny their newfound dependency on the therapist. To be anxious is certainly not "cool," nor does it fit with the belief in personal autonomy that is the hallmark of the teenager's struggle to be on his/her own. These variations on the theme of dependency-autonomy are played out more intensely during the termination phase, and the therapeutic focus should even intensify in anticipation of the ending. If the adolescent does not wish to undo his/her "cool act" and acknowledge the strain of ending the new attachment, it is *unwise to disrupt an adaptive working defense*. But the therapist can help the adolescent acknowledge the progress made and reinforce the role of reflection and understanding and the adolescent's newfound sense of freedom established during the treatment. The opportunity to have a visit at a later date (booster session) if need be can be helpful to some patients.

The reality of the relationship is tacit, but for the sake of the adolescent, is not essential to surging forward in life. Humor is sometimes useful in helping the adolescent to avoid overdramatizing his/her recent dependence and illness. Teens do not take well to overemotional goodbyes, especially boys. Guy-guy or girl-girl kidding is easier to come by than cross-sexual elder child relational sets to effect saying goodbye. Therapists should remember that there have been similar contexts of separations in the adolescent's life that can be reached for. Camp friends, school changes, visiting relatives, and cousins in distant places are all real separations that may help the adolescent to analogize this experience. Goodbye is not necessarily forever, and experiences can be kept in memory.

These varied responses to imminent termination are associated with the developmental stage and the various personality constellations that represent trait-like propensities and unconscious fantasy constellations that refer to earlier unresolved issues largely concerning separation and autonomy. The difference between being a friend (peer) and being friendly and concerned can be distinguished readily at this time to clarify mistaken expectations in our young patients. Moreover, the distinction between being a parent and being a therapist must also be clearly articulated if the child appears to wish to blur these lines. Indeed, therapeutic tolerance and parental patience are both desirable, and each permits the adolescent to discover his/her wishes, aims, and cautions as discrete venues. During termination, the therapist seeks to facilitate a shift from fantasied dependency and realistic holding in the treatment with the therapist as retainer and buffer for anxiety, while preparing the child or adolescent for life with his/her family and/or entrance into adolescent adventures in autonomy and new bonding with peers.

The therapy's recent work, seeking more realistic resolutions, is revisited and made explicit in relation to new feelings, symptoms, longings, and structured fantasies of vulnerability.

4.3.1. The Work of Therapy

The work during this phase concerns the following:

1. *Reflective understanding of prior symptoms* of anxiety employed earlier during the symptomatic phase to better grasp current status and behavior during termination
2. *Regressive solutions*, such as becoming symptomatic again, to new problems that are not adaptive at this phase, with an *emphasis on the child's new ability to reflect on this anachronism*
3. *Healthier and reality-based possibilities offered for conflict resolution* that are in line with developmental stage and coping capacities in line with maturation, less burdened by prior anachronisms
4. The patient's *new and better tolerance for anxiety* that replaces former tendencies to become overwhelmed and/or to regress, which involves more realistic self-assessment and self-modulation and permits a change from seeking dependent solutions rather than autonomous paths

What if the Therapist Has Explored All of These, yet the Child Remains Avoidant?

This rarely happens, but if it does, it is time to start asking the child to explore why he/she hasn't started to take the elevator yet (for example) and what is still holding him/her her back—because the child is well aware that this is like pretending that magic exists every time he/she chooses not to do the frightening or anxiety-provoking thing. *The answer invariably revolves around the child's passive, dependent wishes regarding his/her family (and possibly the therapist, in the transference) and a regressive desire that the therapist (or parent) "do" something*—either force her to stop avoiding (potentially in a masochistically provocative manner, wishing to be "forced" into doing something feared) or, alternatively, in an infantile, passive, magical way, such that the child can deny or avoid his/her own aggressive, assertive wishes by doing what a grown-up says to do. This aspect of the child's transference wishes must be directly articulated.

4.3.2. Case: Fifteen-Year-Old Charlie

Charlie is a 15-year-old high school sophomore who, despite performance anxiety, is enrolled in a performing arts high school. He entered treatment following a panicky feeling and withdrawal that progressed to general anxiety disorder, social anxiety disorder and panic disorder during a summer theater program away from home. He could not go on stage on cue at a group performance. After his anxious arousal, he withdrew to his room.

Anxiety persisted through to the next day when he insisted on calling his mother 100 miles away. The program director suggested his mother take him home, and he left the program.

When home, Charlie seemed somewhat better and less anxious but remained relatively isolated and refused to re-engage with friends. He was very self-critical but demanding of attention and care from his mother. He seemed less interested in talking to his father, a performing musician of some renown.

His family insisted he see a therapist, with whom he engaged cautiously, protesting that it was humiliating to need to be home at age 15. He was ashamed at his clear need for his mother's protection, and he felt like a wimp. During therapy, the central issue that emerged concerned his perfectionism and desire to be applauded and admired. He claimed he was as hard on himself as he felt others were. He slowly began to grasp that his competitive anxiety was tied up in wishing to out-do his father's success at gathering applause. He admitted feeling guilty, too, in gathering in his mother and excluding other family members from her protective attention. She had left the family to pick him up, and he continued to demand her attention at home. He slowly also came to understand that below the anxiety was suppressed anger generated when he could not gain the attention and applause of others.

During the therapy Charlie was able to acknowledge these needs and wishes only to begin to recognize his delight in charming his therapist, making her laugh and creating her as an appreciative audience, but still avoiding friends who were beginning to text and call. Then one day he responded to a text from Becky, a classmate, who wanted him to hang out. That led to further engagements, walks, movies, and even visits with other friends and just hanging out in a group. Nonetheless, during the *termination phase of the therapy* he suddenly grew somber again and complained that the therapist did not seem to be authentic and that she did not laugh as heartily at his jokes and stories. He even pulled back to home, re-enlisting his mother's company, and she called the therapist to register concern about symptom return. The therapist was able to *interpret the threat of losing her as a trigger for the re-engagement around old solutions.* She also reminded Charlie that the *symptoms* seemed to be *replacements for more appropriate, age-related interactions with peers and Becky.* These new experiences gave pleasure yet represented a developmental move away from his mother that was in line with his teen needs and could perhaps be more satisfying than the mental perception of perfection and competitive anger that made up his earlier symptoms. They also considered his prior fantasy of cheering, admiring crowds as a goal that was in fact not likely to be satisfied in immediate reality. He finally tried again to reach out to his new friends and muttered grudgingly during the last encounter, "I guess I don't have to knock 'em dead every time, to have fun!"

4.3.3. Case: Eight-Year-Old Amy

Amy is an eight-year-old girl who presented with separation anxiety disorder. She had been an inhibited toddler who was cautious and clingy. She found it difficult to separate initially when she entered preschool at age three and remained cautious when attending birthdays and larger groups of children. She adapted to school slowly but surely under the guidance of a skilled teacher who gave her extra attention and permitted a more secure separation from her mother. Amy was always obedient and attentive to the school schedule and the structure of daily routines. She soon asked her mother for pre-event assurances that nothing of surprise would ensue. She acquired morning anorexia before school and resisted eating breakfast. At age seven, she started to complain of tummy aches and on two occasions had to be seen at a hospital emergency department to determine whether or not she had a medical condition, such as an acute abdomen or appendicitis. After these events and continued reassurance by her pediatrician, she saw a psychiatrist who diagnosed separation anxiety disorder with tendency toward somatization.

She entered psychotherapy and quickly unloaded her sense of burden, which included disturbing thoughts about danger to mother when she was left with a sitter, problems going to sleep because of worries regarding her younger sister dying in sleep, and more general concerns that she felt "nervous" and that her friends were mean. During the treatment, her worries and anxiety diminished, and her symptoms lifted as she grew to trust her therapist. She felt understood and more confident that she had an ally that matched mother. This developed in the following manner:

At the initial contact with the therapist, Amy was cautious and shyly examined the consulting room while the therapist was silent but welcoming. The therapist did not actively probe Amy's weaknesses and allowed her to initiate conversation/play. Amy was hesitantly monosyllabic until she came on a plush toy dog.

AMY: "Is this yours?"
THERAPIST: "Yes, if you want to you can play with it."
AMY: "It's just like my bed toy Fluffy!"
THERAPIST: "Bed toys are good to have when you are trying to sleep in the dark."
AMY: "I have a nightlight, but I still make my mom sit on my bed until I am asleep." She sighed and added, "But I know she would rather be watching TV, and I get afraid sometimes that she is angry."
THERAPIST: "Well, we have lots of things to talk about, don't we?"

Amy and the therapist further worked to understand her mother's anger and her own anger at her mother as she fantasied abandonment, she felt, because she failed to control her mother as a buffer and safety net. Amy was haunted by unexpressed anger that was defensively transformed to fears that her protector/mother would be in danger, in a relatively common dynamism. It was evident that her anxious but loving mother also was frequently angry because at the height of her child's anxiety, mother seemed overwhelmed and rejecting. Amy's attempts to control her own feelings were extensions of her attempts to control her protector/mother who seemed to become threatening and ready to abandon her.

At the midpoint in therapy when the central dynamism of her worry about abandonment had been exposed, Amy entered the room boasting that she had stopped needing her mother to sit with her at bedtime. The therapist acknowledged her achievement:

THERAPIST: "Good work, that must make you feel so proud!"

AMY: "I still get stomachaches when I have to eat breakfast."

THERAPIST: "I guess you are getting ready to leave Mom in the morning, and that's still scary."

AMY: "It's even worse when she seems angry when I get late and have to eat fast."

THERAPIST: "So your worry is less about leaving than because your Mom doesn't seem happy with you."

AMY: "If she's angry she might not pick me up at school."

THERAPIST: "Has she ever missed?"

AMY: "No"

THERAPIST: "Hey, maybe you worry because you think she knows you are angry when she doesn't OBEY YOU!"

AMY: "I wish I could make her do what I want like magic . . . then I wouldn't worry."

Frequent revisitation to these themes within the therapy aided in dissipating symptoms as Amy began to be more comfortable with not being able to control her mother and to tolerate her own angry feelings.

As *termination approached* and was discussed, Amy feigned indifference to the potential loss of her therapist and joined in the plans for termination. At the same time, her mother reported that she had become more demanding, insisting that she sit at her bedside until she was asleep. She began to dawdle before school and asked for reassurance that mother would pick her up after school in the way she used to before she started therapy. The therapist engaged Amy's curiosity regarding these behaviors and showed her the similarities between her response to termination and her earlier problems regarding fear of losing her mother at times when she had been so angry with her. They reviewed issues concerning her happy state of mind achieved when she was able to join peers in recent months, in contrast to her new clinging and anxious responses to offers from friends versus her dependence on her mother. They reflected on her tendency to experience her anger as anxiety and how she tended to withdraw in unhappiness. She reviewed the comfort of fewer somatic symptoms and her recent ability to tolerate some anxiety and uncertainty and yet to proceed in doing more grown-up things. Amy, for the first time, referred back to her disabling, regressive behaviors as "babyish" and tried to move on. She returned to her more adaptive coping style and left therapy a better friend to her peers and a more mature and comfortable eight-year-old at home with fewer anxiety-ridden episodes of dependence on mother.

4.3.4. Termination Phase: Thirteen-Year-Old Tom

Overview

During the termination phase the previously identified and discussed themes were further worked though and interpreted. Tom became increasingly less anxious and more independent. He was less in need of his mother's constant presence, circulated more independently, and was able to do his work alone. He continued to worry about bad things happening to him, for example, being bitten by a bug and contracting an illness that way.

A new, developmentally appropriate theme that emerged during the termination phase was his budding romantic interests in girls, which he began to share with the therapist, albeit hesitantly and with some embarrassment, which is not unusual for a young teenager like Tom.

He continued to express his desire to want to be like his father, strong and manly, which of course he was not yet, and he expressed indirectly how, on occasions, he felt small and inadequate (see later example).

Tom's positive feelings for the therapist remained and were addressed in the context of the upcoming termination. His defensive pattern of denying upsetting and disappointing feelings surfaced in this context, and the therapist and Tom were able to discuss this as something they had talked about previously that was now happening between them (*transference-focused interpretation*).

The following vignettes illustrate these themes and the psychotherapeutic techniques and interventions employed.

Tom Is Less Socially Avoidant and Makes New Friends

Tom began to study during an afterschool snack with a friend who was a good student and enjoyed studying. The therapist commented on Tom's new behavior by connecting it to his separation anxiety and social avoidance. She said what a good idea it seemed that he was studying more independently and without his mother's help, while at the same time he got to know his friend better. Tom acknowledged this but immediately expressed the *magical worry* of "not wanting to get his hopes up high," wondering whether he just got good grades because it was the end of the term. The therapist commented on his difficulty accepting that things were getting better, but also noted that getting better meant new things were happening and that the unfamiliarity might feel unsettling at times, too.

Tom Wants to Be Like Dad

Tom often talked about "guy activities" with his father, which included attributes of physical strength, such as doing things around the house and garden. It seemed close to his conscious awareness that he wished to be tall and strong like his father, which the therapist gently commented on, by saying he seemed to hope to be like his dad in many ways when he was a grown-up. Tom usually acknowledged this with a slight nod of his head and a forlorn look on his face. By making this comment, the therapist highlighted his positive identification with his father. On a developmental note, this does not imply that Tom may not have had angry or competitive thoughts toward his father at other times, but they were not the focus of his treatment and were not substantially formative in his anxiety symptoms.

One day, Tom continued to express interest in the therapist's office and other peoples' comings and goings and asked the therapist multiple questions. The therapist chose to encourage him to share his thoughts and observations, which led to Tom wondering whether the therapist also saw grown-ups, immediately followed by imagining a big, burly guy sitting where he sat, gesturing the imagined size with his arms. This was followed by him saying that he felt "like a fool" when he couldn't open the door right away when the therapist buzzed him in that day. While at first sight this may look like a non sequitur, the therapist thought this contrast of imaging a strong man in his seat, while feeling foolish himself, revealed how much Tom wished to be more grown-up and how inadequate he actually felt. The therapist chose to not interpret this to Tom and informed this decision by her judgment of *how conscious* this connection was in Tom's mind. The therapist followed the general rule of avoiding the interpretation of unconscious material directly because this can feel jarring to the patient and does not necessarily promote deeper understanding.

Tom Discovers: "Molly's Mean but She Can Be Fun, Too!"

Tom talked about activities with peers, boys and girls, and gave quite detailed accounts about their personalities and their fun activities. He focused on one of the girls, Molly, who he initially described as mean and arrogant, and he then generalized this to other girls, saying all girls were mean. The therapist heard this generalization as a defensive maneuver (if the girls are mean, he does not have to think about whether they are fun and exciting), and she mentioned how much fun he seemed to be having with the other girls and said, "It seems good to know that just because Molly is mean you don't have to avoid all the girls but can have fun with some of them." With this comment, the therapist normalized having fun with girls, an idea Tom had not yet grown comfortable with. This intervention allowed Tom to talk more about what the boys and the girls did together, how they pushed each other into the pool, and he giggled when he described how much fun it was to see them all in jeans and T-shirts, soaking wet. The therapist attempted to explore Tom's curiosity about each other's bodies by saying lightly, "when you're dressed but soaking wet you can kind of see stuff you normally don't see!" to which Tom responded, laughing, "we weren't thinking of that!" Ultimately, Tom talked about a chase between himself and Molly and how she could be a lot of fun, too, and not only arrogant! He seemed excited, yet relieved that such matters could be talked about.

Tom's Reflective Functioning Has Much Improved

By the termination phase, Tom was coming alone to all of his sessions, but he talked about this in a way that sounded a bit forlorn and seemed to emphasize his loneliness. Noticing his affect, the therapist asked Tom how he felt about coming alone, which allowed Tom to explore his feelings about this new behavior and his recent psychological development. He discovered that while he was perfectly capable of coming to the appointment alone, he would like to sometimes be picked up by his mother. Tom felt that the desire to be picked up was maybe "needy," but further discussion allowed him to become accepting of this wish, all the while realizing that the desire for his mother to be there and the absolute need were different kinds of things.

During the penultimate session, the therapist asked Tom what he felt had gotten better and what was still bothering him, to which he replied that his fear of the dark was still there, and it would probably never go away. The therapist encouraged Tom to elaborate but also remarked that he had not brought this up much and recalled how Tom talked about events at night that he found quite exciting. She put Tom's comment into perspective by saying that it seemed he sometimes still had the fear of the dark but not always, and he agreed. Tom said that his mother was also scared of the dark, but she overcame much of it. This was another example of Tom identifying with his mother, the same way he had discovered that he looked at the bright side of things, the way she did. Tom continued by itemizing things and situations that he found scarier than the dark.

A significant improvement for Tom was that he was now able to look more at himself and reflect (improved reflective functioning). For example, he talked about it being "odd" that he liked scary movies that are all about the dark and wondered what this might mean. The therapist offered as an explanation that this might be the case because in the movie it is not *his* fear and the scary stuff is "outside of him." This then led to Tom talking about how he liked to scare others, in particular girls, "one to two years ago." He described some of his pranks and how he had a friend sit on his shoulder so that he would seem scarier because he was taller. This was an example of *turning passive into active*, scaring others rather than being scared himself, but also an expression of how the experiences of being excited and being scared felt connected for him. He explained that he was not doing this stuff as much since it stopped working because "the girls are not as gullible." The therapist interpreted that Tom might also have less of a need to scare them because *he* was less scared nowadays.

Tom talked about a friend who got a bug bite and the bug had a "disease." He said it in a way that sounded somber, and the therapist responded to his affect, asking whether he was worried, too? Tom said that he was, but that after all it was not very likely that the same bug would come back and bite him and that therefore there was not so much reason to worry. Tom applied a somewhat immature pseudo-logic here by thinking only about the same bug who bit his friend, but it did serve its purpose, which was to help him with his anxiety over getting an illness from the bug, and his fears were not as much informed by his magical thinking as they had been in the past.

Tom "Forgot" That Treatment Will End Soon and Then Plans a Party for the Last Session

Tom continued to express his thoughts about the therapist's office space and office mates, and the therapist acknowledged his curiosity as well as his skill for keen observation, which included new "discoveries" he made, such as about individuals he saw in the waiting area, who seemed to know whom, and so forth. Of note, many of Tom's comments about the therapist were indirect, in that they often focused on material things and other people in the office. This was a *displaced* expression of a positive transference (and possibly romantic interest) that Tom was more comfortable with than a more direct expression of affection or toleration of impending loss. The therapist acknowledged Tom's observations to foster his *increasing comfort with the contents of his mind*. The therapist then connected these themes to the upcoming termination by commenting that it might be hard to finish sometime soon because he so much liked coming now. This triggered a surprise reaction in Tom who had "forgotten" that treatment would end soon, which was immediately followed by plans for an over-the-top, circus-like party for his last session. This was clearly a defense against the impending sadness about the loss of the relationship with the therapist, and she said to Tom that it seemed easier to talk about a party than his having forgotten the ending and his disappointment about treatment ending soon. The therapist and Tom talked more about his avoidance of sadness and upsetting feelings by being overly excited and funny.

Tom shared the following fantasy about the upcoming termination: while he was doing his work independently now, he sometimes felt overwhelmed by the amount and imagined staying over in the therapist's office, doing his homework there. He imagined that he would even stay once the next patient came in and the therapist would say to that person that he was just imagining Tom being there. Tom continued, saying that he would hide in the closet. The therapist interpreted that with termination coming so soon, Tom seemed to be thinking about ways to spend more time in her office and also about how he and the therapist would have a secret together, him hiding in the closet.

For the first time, Tom took a taxi alone on his way to his final session and refrained from calling his mother to ask how much to tip the driver and decided by himself. He proudly reported this to the therapist, who shared his happiness and commented on Tom trying out something new as his treatment was ending. Tom could finally talk in limited ways about his feelings about the ending of the treatment and said that the idea of not coming anymore to his twice-weekly sessions felt "weird" and that he felt like he had been coming to see the therapist for years. He imagined seeing the therapist around the neighborhood, which was a way to make the termination less real and painful.

Thirteen-year-old Tom who had initially presented with a long history of social phobia, and separation anxiety disorder lost his anxiety diagnoses when ADIS he was reassessed at the time treatment ended (social phobia 1/8, separation anxiety disorder 2/8, dysthymic disorder 4/8). Gains were maintained at six months' follow-up and his dysthymia had improved as well. He functioned at a much improved adaptive level relatively free of anxiety.

4.4. Summary

This chapter provides a guide to the opening, middle, and termination phases of CAPP. The opening phase serves to obtain the history of the symptoms, to establish a therapeutic alliance with the youth and his/her parents, and to identify core psychological dynamisms that contribute to the child's anxieties. From the outset, the therapist pays attention to the beginning transference development, as well as countertransference reactions, which, for example, in anxious children can include feeling the need to quickly assuage patients' distress. The therapist addresses maladaptive behavioral patterns early but sensitively and interprets defenses before addressing conscious or unconscious fantasies.

During the middle phase, the therapist and patient collaboratively understand the previously identified central psychological conflicts and core dynamisms as they pertain to anxiety symptoms. As new material emerges, adjustments to the initial formulation can be made. The therapist interprets defense mechanisms and attends to the deepening transference to the therapist. The developing understanding of the meaning of the anxiety symptoms results in a progressive improvement in reflective functioning, which is followed by improved functioning. Multiple examples of therapeutic interactions are given in the text.

The termination phase describes how the ending of treatment presents a unique opportunity to review psychological and symptomatic changes that have occurred and also to revisit earlier symptoms, in particular in the context of the common rearousal of symptoms in which separation conflicts are now experienced with the therapist in the transference. New venturesome behaviors that point toward adaptive and sensible autonomy-seeking are encouraged, without the burden of previous maladaptive restrictions.

The authors demonstrate through clinical examples that CAPP can accomplish the following:

- Reduce anxiety symptoms by articulating anxious fantasies in words rather than symptoms or actions and developing an understanding of the emotional meaning of symptoms and associated behaviors
- Enhance the child's skill of reflection and self-observation of one's own and others' motivations, ideas, and behaviors, with the expectation of continued use after treatment ends (improvement in symptom-specific reflective functioning)
- Diminish children's use of avoidance, age-inappropriate dependence and rigidity by helping them to see that underlying emotions such as guilt, shame, and anger, as well as wishes and desires that seem unacceptable, can be tolerated and understood
- Understand fantasies and compelling emotional significance surrounding the anxiety symptoms, which reduces symptoms' magical qualities and powerful impact on the child by articulating personal meanings in language

References

1. Makari, G., & Shapiro, T. (1993). On psychoanalytic listening: Language and unconscious communication. *Journal of the American Psychiatric Association, 41*, 991–1020.

2. Main, M., & Goldwyn, R. (1994). *Adult attachment rating and classification system* (Manual in draft, Version 6.0). Unpublished Manuscript, University of California at Berkeley.

3. American Psychiatric Association. (1994). *Diagnostic and statistical manual of mental disorders* (4th ed.). Washington, DC: American Psychiatric Press.

4. Silverman, W. K., & Albano, A. M. (2004). *Anxiety Disorders Interview Schedule (ADIS-IV): Child and Parent Version*. New York, NY: Oxford University Press and Graywind Publications.

5

Including Parents of Children and Adolescents in Dynamic Psychotherapy of Anxiety

5.1. Theory and Clinical Issues

Because humans require active and prolonged caretaking of relatively dependent and immature children, parents serve as stewards and buffers to the external world. During these early years before puberty, children often do not personally acknowledge their distress or unhappiness. Indeed, the parent most often is the family member to seek professional help, noticing the child's behavioral anxiety, irritability, anger, clinging, or isolation: the parents, often the mother or her substitute, bring the child to a professional and serves as the initial informant. As adolescence emerges, he/she may not be willing to show feelings that are embarrassing because the feelings may be experienced as child-like and may instead alert a parent by behavioral manifestations of anxiety: avoidance, withdrawal, irritability, or panicky behavior when asked to do things that arouse anxiety. Furthermore, some anxious children whose developmental level would suggest better autonomy, can tantrum and panic, embarrassing parents and exposing their inability to modulate their anxious child (1).

This chapter addresses the following questions about balancing parental involvement in CAPP: When the diagnosis and treatment plan are in place, how does the dynamic therapist consider parents? What will be the parents' role in the treatment? How are parents kept engaged while exploration with the child proceeds? How does the therapy deal with parents who demonstrate a need to be included in the new therapeutic dyadic relationship? How does the therapist ensure parental cooperation? When should the therapist see the parents again after treatment has begun, and what are insistent indicators that parents should be seen? In short, parents must be included in the therapeutic process in some manner if the therapy is to survive, which necessarily involves gaining parental cooperation.

Initially, the parents serve as informants regarding symptoms, signs, and adaptation at home, at school, and in the exercise of tasks of daily living. They provide insight into home life, expectations, and educational and disciplinary beliefs. The various relationships with each parent and sibling must be well explored from the parental perspective as a way of improving understanding of the child's state of mind and the degree to which the family environment does or does not support maturation and symptom formation. In addition, parents provide information regarding developmental landmarks and temperamental tendencies and expose the triggers that play a role in anxiety onset. The therapist learns from parents about parental conflicts and changes in family function, about crises and school reports, and about breeches with friends and recent separations. Parents provide the rich array of familial and cultural backdrops to be considered, including recent moves, living circumstances, and neighborhood and safety. Parents also offer their view on caution or license for autonomy as well as their estimate of trust in the child's capacity for self-modulation. Finally, the interview should reveal the nonexplicit array of family allegiances and conflicts to which the child adapts (2, 3).

After parents provide these vital stories, they must also be made to feel confident that the therapist can be trusted to handle their child with respect and competence so that they can allow a new relationship that mostly excludes their (understandably) anxious eyes and ears. Some parents seem to feel the need to know how things are going in the child's psychotherapy or become worried as symptoms accentuate or improve or give rise to changes in home expectations that affect the usual family equilibrium. Under the latter circumstances, the therapist may invite the parents into the office for a mid-course visit. Throughout the therapy, parents should feel able to contact the therapist under any circumstances that they feel is urgent.

In the case of adolescent patients, for whom confidentiality is often a central concern, it is recommended to have such meetings including teenage patient and one or both parents together to help facilitate better communication and greater autonomy in the teen. This open confrontation also helps convince the teen that his/her privacy has been respected and that the parents can be trusted to support the treatment relationship.

It is essential to determine to what degree the parents inadvertently collude with or encourage the child's anxiety symptoms, thereby perpetuating or aggravating the expression of anxiety. How punitive or permissive and indulgent are they? Can they tolerate the child's expressing distress at all? Where does this child fit into the family? To what extent are the anxiety symptoms a manifestation of a socially reinforced role, maybe through sibship dynamics? To what extent is the family triangulated with tendencies toward alliances that are perpetuated by long habit and rigid affections and selectively hostile ties? The therapist attempts to articulate unsaid alliances that may be at work that support the perpetuation of symptoms. Such interventions are focused on the plight of the child and not intended as family interventions. They are educative in nature but can have a positive therapeutic effect.

In some instances, when inadvertent or unconscious reinforcement of symptoms is suspected, the therapist may wish to make inquiries of the parent to attempt to determine unconscious motives for participating in bed sharing, for example, with the anxious child, which necessarily encourages regression. In other instances of hostile and even violent family discord, parents might have to be invited to explore the roots of their unrest, and the therapist may need to indicate that the adolescent's symptoms lack the support to change within certain home conditions, such as those in which chronic fighting has become a norm. Relationships between parents and children are complicated and multifaceted. Anxiety in a child can become a trigger for unrest, disappointment, and fear of future failure in the family. Any or all of these factors may be at work in maintaining the child's symptoms and can prevent functional and symptomatic improvement.

It is important that the therapist avoid "analyzing" the parent, or becoming the parent's therapist in any way. In a time-limited psychotherapy treatment with a child, the therapist is forging a bond that by design will be broken soon and that must be respected by gearing the therapy toward the child's developmental capacities after treatment without the therapeutic support and with a goal of shifting back to the available family support as the treatment comes to an end (4).

Termination is often very productive but can be a challenging time in CAPP, when the child revisits his/her personal dynamisms as separation from the therapist looms imminent. Termination and the complex emotional backdrop that this process imports into CAPP is covered in depth in Chapter 4. For parents, this may require a parental visit so that the parents do not, unwittingly, escalate the child's anxiety level further with their own worries that the treatment might not "work" or that their child's improvement may be tied to dependence on a therapist. It can be complicated for parents to understand that termination can be a time of symptomatic regression because the termination process arouses renewed anxiety in their youngster. Revisiting with parents at termination is sometimes indicated, and a psycho-educational meeting can help to further parents' understanding of their child's (now much improved) symptomatic anxieties.

In such pre-termination parental meetings, it can be helpful to remind parents of the child's improvements over the course of the therapy. This intervention helps to calm parents and decrease levels of ambient anxiety, and it underscores and encourages parental support of positive therapeutic outcomes (see the case example of Jimmy presented later). During such a visit, the therapist can also inquire how the parents view the patient's behavior, how they have been adapting to the changes they have observed, and whether there are new developmental thrusts toward independence and autonomy and fewer anxiety outbursts and avoidance behaviors.

5.1.1. Specific Aspects of Working With Parents of Young Children

Developmentally younger children are, by necessity, dependent on their families and not autonomous. Children are brought by their concerned parents who are their guardians and stewards. We cannot assume that a parent's reasons for engagement in therapy are fully understood by the child. Nor would we expect that parents would support the engagement if they thought their aims were at odds with the aims of the treatment. Parents may frame their complaints differently than the therapist formulates the problems, such as when parents' motivation for seeking therapy might be a wish that their child would behave and not be fearful or inhibited, while the therapist might recognize the therapeutic goal and focus of resolving internal conflicts that would give the child more freedom to become adaptive to his/her school and home. While the family is educated about the importance of the child's privacy, anxious parents particularly often desire a "peephole" into their child's emotional life and can fear they might be replaced or discarded as the child develops too close of a trusting relationship with the therapist. This issue is of vibrant concern to parents with anxious attachments, who form a large proportion of the parents of anxious child patients. To the contrary, in the apparently opposite set of dynamisms, therapists who begin to gather that the parent is "dumping" the management of their child's anxieties should quickly repeat the bargain of the therapy and reject any implied surrogacy that eschews respect for parental concern, cooperation, and participation (5).

5.1.2. Specific Aspects of Working With Parents of Adolescents

Working with parents of adolescents presents challenges because of the patient's emerging autonomy and blossoming need for privacy, whether the patient articulates these concerns or not. Recommendations vary as to whether parents of teenagers should be included in any aspect of therapy after the adolescent has reached ages 15 to 17, but we reserve this option in CAPP if the adolescent's maturity is flagging and/or deviance and/or poor social adaptation or unexpected changes emerge that require closer and collaborative vigilance because age alone does not correspond to maturational competence. In time-limited CAPP, these are common occurrences. The therapist may wish to keep the parents closer and more involved in the treatment of the relatively immature teenager, using them as collaborative associates in the therapy. Meetings with parents of teens had best be aboveboard: the teen may wish to be present to ascertain and secure the promise of privacy (6).

Three case examples follow: seven-year-old Wendy, seven-year-old Annie, and 13-year-old Jimmy.

5.2. Cases

5.2.1. Seven-Year-Old Wendy: Engaging and Supporting the Parents

Wendy, an anxious seven-year-old who won't separate from a parent at school, refuses breakfast, and has daily tantrums as she leaves home, is brought in by her parents. Wendy becomes argumentative when dressing in choosing her clothes. Her mother has the lion's share of the problem because her father leaves early for work and arrives home just as Wendy is about to go to bed.

The following dialogue is taken from the first appointment with the parents.

MOTHER: I am at my wits' end. I get so frantic when she is anxious that I lash out at her and shout.

FATHER: That just makes things worse.

MOTHER: You think I don't know that? You are never there anyway and are no help.

THERAPIST: So you feel you have no one to share the burden with.

MOTHER: You bet, and then I fight with him about her, and he has no ideas except that "it will go away."

FATHER: I know that you are suffering, but she is scared.

MOTHER: Yeah, and she suffers, too, and you go scot-free to work.

THERAPIST: You mention she suffers?

MOTHER: Yeah, she is so panicky and worries all the time. I worry she can't concentrate and get her work done.

THERAPIST: No doubt, but it sounds like both of you are also very upset.

MOTHER: I feel so for her. I've been there myself, and it's so hard when she has no one to lean on who is in charge.

FATHER: I could be, if you weren't so angry at me, as if I did it to her.

THERAPIST: So there is no calm place or shoulder to lean on in all the house. Nonetheless, she seems to want to be at home and not at school.

MOTHER: That's because she's scared.

THERAPIST: Is there anything at school that's scary?

MOTHER: I guess not—maybe her thoughts.

THERAPIST: Oh! Tell me what you know about her thoughts?

MOTHER: I guess whether I'm all right, am I distraught or sick.

THERAPIST: I know you get distraught, but sick?

MOTHER: I complain a lot.

FATHER: She has stomachaches frequently, and the doctor doesn't seem to be of help.

THERAPIST: I guess you are both wondering if I can be of help.

MOTHER: I don't want to believe that, otherwise or I'm sunk.

THERAPIST: Sunk?

MOTHER: Yeah, without a lifeboat.

THERAPIST: So I guess as your lifeboat I shouldn't be panicky.

MOTHER: That would be nice.

THERAPIST: I guess it would be. It sounds like it would be good if Wendy could believe you were safe like a lifeboat, she might be able to trust more.

MOTHER: Trust more?

THERAPIST: Yes—be able to use you as a lifeline and trust that you were there for her.

MOTHER: Then she could believe I'm a support and not just as upset as she is?

In this brief encounter, we see a parallel process emerging rapidly between the therapist and mother's expectations and wishes in establishing this new therapeutic relationship for Wendy, and the mother and daughter's expectations and wishes from her mother. This provides an opportunity to bring the behaviors that create the climate for symptom expression to active awareness for the mother.

5.2.2. Seven-Year-Old Annie: Treatment During a Crisis

Annie, a seven-year-old, was engaged in treatment during the tumultuous early stages of what was to end in parental divorce. While the parents had stopped bickering and were now seeking independent lives while still living together, tensions still ran high. Father was out of the home many more evenings, and weekends were spent with each parent in separate outings. The maternal grandmother was called in to baby-sit more frequently. The tension at home was crackling.

The therapist realized that Annie had privy to more facts than the parents knew. She also was more curious about the new arrangements, and in her therapy, she played repeatedly about themes of abandonment, anger, helplessness, and abortive rescue by external superheroes.

During the course of CAPP the therapist decided that it seemed wise in this complex system to see the parents more frequently to work with them on their view of what Annie knew and to work with them on the repercussions of secrecy and tension at home in order to help them to try and minimize these problems. It was possible to offer the child a buffer during treatment against abandonment while the parents gradually could feel secure enough to relax the secrecy about their evolving separation and approach the pending separation more directly so as to consider their child's fears and offer corrective reassurances bolstered by some changes. They were able to assure Annie that although they were indeed planning to live apart, they would be steadfast in their love and protection toward her. The therapy also provided Annie with continuity during the uncertain period of emotional tension and unpredictability.

5.2.3. Thirteen-Year-Old Jimmy: "Do We Like This 'New' Jimmy?"

Jimmy was approaching age 14 as his treatment was ending. He no longer asked repeated unnecessary questions, was sleeping in his own bed, had stopped dawdling in the morning, and was arriving on time to school. However, he had become more defiant and aggressive at home, contradicting his parents on the most trivial suggestions and arguing more frequently with his younger sibling about his rights as an older brother. The parents were uneasy with his new assertiveness and called the therapist frequently about how to address this "new Jimmy." They were not sure they liked this new version of their son any better than the passive but sweet and anxious "prior version."

The parents were invited into the therapist's office to discuss Jimmy's new developmental thrust toward autonomy that adolescence—and the psychotherapy—had fostered.

BOX 5.1 Including Parents in Treatment

- Parent or surrogate is essential to optimal maturation
- Parent is the usual first informant regarding chief complaint, context, and family structure
- Parents' interests must be attended for treatment to proceed and succeed
- Therapist should not ally with child or adolescent solely, unless abuse or neglect is detected
- Outcome depends on triadic change: patient, parent (tolerating and adapting to change in the child), and therapist

The parents were given an opportunity to describe what they thought had happened to Jimmy and appeared peeved that the therapist might have been fostering parental criticism and random autonomy provocation. The therapist offered an alternative perspective: that Jimmy had been sitting anxiously on his venturesome side and had suppressed his desire to shine and be a player among his peers because of elements of his anxious attachment to his parents. The therapist offered the parents some suggestions involving becoming more tolerant of their own anxiety regarding Jimmy's new assertiveness and what seemed to be disrespect. The therapist encouraged the parents to be more accepting of Jimmy's new ability to verbalize his desires, and he suggested that they try to develop some sense of humor about some of Jimmy's outbursts. The therapist reassured the parents that Jimmy would not become the monster that they feared and was more likely to be happier and even more attached in a healthier way if they permitted some room for him to express himself and engage his parents in conversation about his life. This youngster did not balk at the therapist's seeing his parents and even felt validated and proceeded uneventfully to termination.

5.3. Summary

Parents or a parent surrogate is essential for child and adolescent survival (Box 5.1). The parent serves as a buffer, mediating with the world until the individuation process is as nearly complete as possible (7). Psychological readiness is not always in lockstep with physical maturation. In view of this biological universal, parents are an essential participant in any therapy—as historians, context providers, and as necessary coparticipants and context informants—because they help the therapeutic aim.

References

1. Shapiro, T. (2003). Diagnosis and diagnostic formulation. In Wiener J. & Dulcan, M. (Eds.), *Textbook of child and adolescent psychiatry* (3rd ed., pp. 175–184). Washington, DC: American Psychiatric Press.
2. Keaney, B. P. (1985). *Mind in therapy: Constructing systemic family therapies.* New York, NY: Basic Books.
3. Haley, J. (1968). *Techniques of family therapy.* New York, NY: Basic Books.

4. Mc Dermott, J. (1974). The undeclared war between child psychiatry and family therapy. *American Journal of Child Psychiatry, 13*, 422–436.

5. Tsiantis, J., Boethious, S. B., Horne, A., & Hallefors, B. (Eds). (2000). *Work with parents: Psychoanalytic psychotherapy with children and adolescents.* London, UK: Karnac.

6. Blos, P. (1967). The second individuation process. *Psychoanalytic Study of the Child, 22*, 162–186.

7. Bowlby, J. (1958). The nature of the child's tie to his mother. *International Journal of Psychoanalysis 39*, 350–373.

The Anxiety Disorders

CAPP has been studied in children and adolescents aged seven to 16 with primary *Diagnostic and Statistical Manual of Mental Disorders, fourth edition* (DSM-IV) generalized anxiety disorder (GAD), separation anxiety disorder, and social anxiety disorder (social phobia) diagnoses. Panic disorder, agoraphobia with or without comorbid major depression, and posttraumatic stress disorder (PTSD) were frequent comorbidities. The following sections will describe symptoms, signs, diagnostic criteria, salient psychodynamic factors, and treatment techniques. The reader is referred to Table 6.1, which summarizes psychodynamic theory, target symptoms, and treatment strategies, followed by specific clinical approaches, rounding out variations of core fantasies and changes in techniques expected for each variant of the anxiety disorders.

Case examples for each disorder will be offered.

6.1. Generalized Anxiety Disorder With Case Vignette

6.1.1. Symptoms, Signs, and Diagnostic Considerations

GAD was first introduced into the child and adolescent psychiatric diagnostic nomenclature with DSM-IV (1). Before DSM-IV, GAD was considered a condition affecting individuals over age 18, and children and teens with comparable symptoms were diagnosed with overanxious disorder of childhood. The collapsing of the adult and child diagnoses into the same diagnostic categorical criteria reflects recognition that these are continuous conditions rather than distinct entities.

Anxiety in children has been described as early as the 18th century when Genevan philosopher Jean-Jacques Rousseau and English philosopher John Locke recommended treatment of "irrational fears" in children (2). Freud's 1895 diagnostic features of "anxiety neurosis" share features of GAD (3, 4), in addition to features of panic disorder.

TABLE 6.1 **Relationship Between Dynamic Theory and Interventions for Anxiety in CAPP**

Anxiety Disorder/Symptoms and Features	Dynamic Theory in CAPP	Target Symptoms and CAPP Strategies
Social anxiety disorder (social phobia)	Self-consciousness and fears of embarrassment are linked to conflicted wishes to outshine others and are laced with guilt and self-punishment; such competition feels laden with unacceptable destructive aggression.	Explore defenses against wishes to stand out; conflicted patients' overly critical evaluation of others is an entrée to connections with uncomfortable competitive wishes and conflicted, unacceptable aggression. This raises symptom-specific reflective functioning (SSRF).
Generalized anxiety disorder (GAD)	Inability to relax and need to maintain constant vigilance arises from conflicts related to frightening personal meanings that threaten to arise in consciousness; passive sexual and aggressive wishes are triggered by daily experiences and feel overwhelming; experienced anxiety cannot be mastered by usual mental work.	Focus on terror of internal urges, including aggression and desire for autonomy. Emerging fantasies are actively connected with symptoms and persistence of anxiety. This raises SSRF.
Separation anxiety disorder	Developmentally inappropriate separation distress arises from conflict between normal strivings for autonomy and concerns about hurting/abandoning the emotionally needed parent. Clinging leads to anger at parent and self, stemming from dim awareness of its out-of-phase regressive significance. Fears of separation *per force* emerge in the transference, making termination a key time to address this problem.	Explore transference relationship, an emotionally vibrant paradigm for understanding and altering separation fears. Emotional significance of termination is a central topic of the final third of treatment. This raises SSRF.
Anxiety about establishing age-appropriate autonomy (a common feature of social anxiety disorder, separation anxiety disorder, and generalized anxiety disorder)	Conflicts and fears about autonomy emerge in the transference. Assertiveness is perceived as destructive anger that can interfere with attachment relationships. The conflict arouses anxiety with fears of abandonment.	CAPP focus on transference highlights conflicts about autonomy, especially as incorporated into fantasies of bodily harm and inadequacy and experienced as bodily anxiety and symptoms.
Comorbid major depression (when present)	Conflicted aggression leads to guilt and negative self-evaluation, depressive symptoms, and somatic anxiety.	CAPP focus on conflicted aggression detoxifies it, and helps patient redirect it, leading to improved autonomous function and greater assertion. It mitigates guilt, with improvement in autonomy, and negative views of self improve.
(Seemingly) out-of-the blue panic attacks	Panic attacks arise from specific unconscious conflicts/fantasies that carry symbolic meaning. As patient begins to grasp this symbolic meaning, the panic disappears.	Focus on emotional significance of panic: identify and interpret specific psychological meaning of physical symptoms. Explore and interpret emotional significance of triggers. Help patients to understand their internal emotional states. This raises SSRF.

TABLE 6.1 **Continued**

Anxiety Disorder/Symptoms and Features	Dynamic Theory in CAPP	Target Symptoms and CAPP Strategies
Agoraphobia	Agoraphobia is an unconscious way of controlling attachment figures, while retaining a nonthreatening, age-inappropriate childish stance that serves to deny aggression.	Explore management of rage at attachment figures. Interpret need to avoid aggression, with anger expressed as dependent and controlling anxious neediness. Openly discuss, normalize, and detoxify rage. Focus on how agoraphobia and dependence on phobic companions maintains an age-inappropriate childish stance. Agoraphobic fantasies involve fantasies of walled-off danger zones and also artificially magical "safe" zones. This should be emphasized.

There is increasing evidence that biological, constitutional, familial, developmental, psychological, environmental (5), and psychodynamic conflicts contribute to the phenomenological presentation of GAD (4). The gender ratio is approximately equal until adolescence, after which females predominate. The disorder can appear at any age, but there is an increased onset with advancing age, especially in females after the onset of puberty. There is lack of diagnostic stability, and GAD can emerge from other anxiety disorders or transform into other anxiety disorders. In addition, there are significant overlaps with other anxiety disorders and high rates of comorbidity. About 50% of affected children show comorbid separation anxiety disorder, phobic disorders, major depression, mood disorders, and attention deficit disorder (4, 6).

GAD has significant impact on children's and families' lives and can interfere with successful completion of necessary developmental accomplishments. It affects interpersonal relationships within the family and with peers, academic functioning, and overall happiness and satisfaction.

GAD is defined in DSM-5 (7) as "excessive anxiety and worry (apprehensive expectation), occurring more days than not for at least 6 months, about a number of events or activities . . . ", "The person finds it difficult to control the worry", and the worry is accompanied by restlessness, fatigue, difficulty concentrating, irritability, muscle tension, and insomnia (three symptoms required for adults, one for children). The overlapping dynamics of the anxiety syndromes in children and adolescents may help in treatment of the comorbidity of GAD, separation anxiety disorder, and social anxiety disorder and in identifying approaches to diminishing common sets of symptoms.

6.1.2. Psychodynamic Factors and Conflicts

Children and teens with GAD tend to have the fantasy that they must maintain control or be vigilant at all times, or else catastrophe will result. This hypervigilant state can develop from a persistent fear of the conscious emergence of unacceptable feelings and fantasies and an associated fear of loss of control. In GAD, psychological defense mechanisms are relatively ineffective at neutralizing or disguising unconscious wishes, leading to a feeling of ongoing threat and struggle with unacceptable feelings and fantasies. Rather than denying upsetting feelings altogether, these patients experience persistent jealous or angry feelings that frighten them. Alternatively, somatization and worry may be operating as defenses against unacceptable feelings and fantasies. Chronic worrying can also emerge in response to early relationships that come to form an internal psychological template in which attachments are experienced as fragile or easily disrupted. The developmental experiences of GAD patients can trigger feelings of rejection, potential loss, anger, and a sense of needing to protect the caregiver to maintain the relationship (8). Such responses frequently occur in children of depressed mothers. Traumatic events can heighten the sense of the need for hypervigilance. The need for control, fears of disruption to attachment relationships, and defenses against important emotional cues have an adverse impact on current interpersonal relationships, exacerbating chronic worries.

Researchers from various backgrounds have arrived at conclusions that overlap with this psychodynamic formulation (8, 9). *Worry is employed as a less than adaptive, somewhat magical attempt to regulate events and emotions.* As a result of these pressures, these patients lack access to interpersonal cues because of constant preoccupations, leading to greater problems in their relationships. Cassidy et al. (9) suggest that these difficulties develop from insecure attachment, leading to problems in affect regulation and fears about dangers in interpersonal relationships. They found evidence of insecure attachment in GAD patients, including a feeling that they need to take care of their parents. These persistent fears and emotional difficulties lead to ineffective attempts to obtain security from others.

6.1.3. Treatment: Transdiagnostic Techniques and Specific Adaptations

As in other symptomatically targeted psychodynamic approaches to anxiety disorders, the therapist explores the content of the patient's specific worries, how they are experienced, and the associated thoughts and the particular sense of dread. The goal of the inquiry is to determine the particular threatening—at least partially—unconscious fantasies that the child is attempting to manage or displace, in an effort to make his/her emotional reactions more understandable. Early life relationships and traumatic experiences are investigated to determine the experiential basis of the child's view of the world as unsafe. The therapist works with the child/adolescent to identify the sources of the threat of loss of control if vigilance is not maintained at all times. Precipitants of a worsening of GAD symptoms are actively explored, including an exploration of times and interpersonal circumstances in which the anxiety symptoms intensify. The therapist identifies and explores defenses, including somatization, which is often triggered when intrapsychic conflicts are not admissible to consciousness.

Further clues can be obtained from experiences of anxiety in the transference. The therapy provides a safe atmosphere in which frightening unconscious wishes and conflicts can emerge, including those the child may experience about the therapist, and can be rendered less threatening. However, even in this "safe" atmosphere, patients with GAD can experience a sense of threat in the therapeutic relationship. The experience of this threat provides an opportunity to examine more directly the patient's catastrophic fears of loss of control. Issues of separation and attachment, addressed throughout therapy, intensify and can be highlighted during the termination process.

As an outline or paradigm of the various sorts of underlying fantasies, Freud's list of developmental triggers of danger (10), such as fear of helplessness, fears of separation from close attachment figures, fears of bodily harm, and internalized superego (moral values) discordance, is relevant.

6.1.4. Case: Seven-Year-Old Gary

Gary's mother described her seven-year-old first-grader as a constant worrier who followed her around the apartment "as though his life depended on me." She allowed that she herself was an anxious woman and that she saw a replica of herself in her son and felt guilty for every separation. Gary was an inhibited and shy toddler, and she had avoided sending him to preschool, only to find that his separation anxiety at kindergarten necessitated her planned attendance with him for a longer span than she had expected. He finally adapted and now attended first grade with relative ease, but she had a great deal of difficulty getting him out the door in the morning. He dawdled and seemed uninterested in breakfast, complaining of tummy aches and demanding that she take him to the door of his classroom.

When in school, he seemed to take to his teacher and made a few friends with whom he exchanged Pokémon cards and talked during recess. Gary anxiously anticipated his mother's appearance at school dismissal, frequently asking his teacher if she thought his mother would be there. His mother often took him for a snack after school, and they shopped sometimes. Gary began his almost ritualized litany of questions concerning whether mom and dad would be "going out" and who would babysit for him and his younger sister. He did well at school and was dutiful about getting his brief homework done. About twice weekly he had outbursts at his father or mother, shouting they were unfair because they permitted his younger sister to go to sleep at the same bedtime as his, or that she was been given more dessert than him.

He seemed to worry a great deal about his mother's safety when she was to leave him. He also confessed to his mother that he had recurrent concerns that their home was not burglarproof and that his bedroom window was close to a fire escape, permitting entry. These worries often kept him up at night even though he had permission to read himself to sleep and keep a nightlight. He wakened at least three times a week and wandered into his parents' bedroom. They encouraged return to his own bed, but he preferred to slip into their bed near his mother. Overall, he carried on his hobbies, drawing cartoon characters and joining his friends, but he did not accept sleepover invitations.

Gary was capable of having fun and enjoyed the times when he was free of anxiety and intermittent stomachaches. However, the anxious ruminations often interrupted play dates or family outings and would spoil his free time. He seemed aware that some of his worries were "silly," but he claimed not to be able to help it and became whiney and fidgety and restless. He often seemed to be embarrassed because he recognized he was being "like a baby." Gary's excellent access to his fantasy life, including his rescue fantasies, could be easily transformed for therapeutic effect into a narrative of healthier life goals. He also carried a strong inner awareness of his rich array of fantasies, some of which he could turn to narrative advantage when not preoccupied.

References

1. American Psychiatric Association. (1994). *Diagnostic criteria from diagnostic and statistical manual of mental disorders* (4th ed.). Washington, DC: American Psychiatric Press.
2. McDermott, J., Werry, J., Petti, T., Combrinck-Graham, L., & Char, W. (1989). Anxiety disorders of childhood or adolescence. In T. Karasu (Ed.), *Treatment of psychiatric disorders: A task force report of the American Psychiatric Association* (Vol. 1, pp. 401–443). Washington, DC: American Psychiatric Publishing.
3. Freud, S. (1895). *On the grounds for detaching a particular syndrome from neurasthenia under the description "anxiety neurosis"* (Standard ed. 3, pp. 85–115). London, UK: Hogarth Press.
4. Stine, J. (1997). Overanxious disorder of childhood. In: J. D. Noshpitz, P. F. Kernberg, & J. R. Bemporad (Eds.), *Handbook of child and adolescent psychiatry* (Vol. 2, pp. 530–556). New York, NY: Wiley and Sons.
5. Aktar, E., Nikolic, M., & Boegels, S. M. (2017). Environmental transmission of generalized anxiety disorder from parents to children: Worries, experiential avoidance, and intolerance of uncertainty. *Dialogues in Clinical Neuroscience, 19*(2), 137–147.
6. Last, C. G., Herson, M., Kazdin, A. E., Francis, G., & Grubb, H. J. (1987). Psychiatric illness in the mothers of anxious children. *American Journal of Psychiatry, 144*, 1580–1583.
7. American Psychiatric Association. (2013). *Diagnostic criteria from diagnostic and statistical manual of mental disorders* (5th ed.). Washington, DC: American Psychiatric Press.
8. Crits-Christoph, P., Crits-Christoph, K., Wolf-Palacio, D., Fichter, M., & Rudick, D. (1995). Brief supportive-expressive psychodynamic therapy for generalized anxiety disorder. In: J. P. Barber & P. Crits-Christoph (Eds.), *Dynamic therapies for psychiatric disorders (Axis I)* (pp. 43–83). New York, NY: Basic Books.
9. Cassidy, J., Lichtenstein-Phelps, J., Sibrava, N. J., Thomas, C. L. Jr., & Borkovec, T. D. (2009). Generalized anxiety disorder: Connections with self-reported attachment. *Behavior Therapy, 40*, 23–38.
10. Freud, S. (1923). *The ego and the id* (Standard ed. 19, pp. 1–66). London, UK: Hogarth Press.

6.2. Social Anxiety Disorder With Case Vignette

6.2.1. Symptoms, Signs, and Diagnostic Considerations

Diagnosis of social anxiety disorder in children and adolescents requires the same cluster of symptoms (1) that are used to characterize the adult disorder, including persistent anxiety symptoms for six months. Marked fear and/or anxiety should be present in one or more social situations, which include scrutiny by others: in conversation, meeting others, being observed, or performing. The child or adolescent has the tendency to evaluate the meeting negatively in anticipation, describing embarrassment, humiliation, and rejection that promote anxiety, withdrawal, freezing, and even tears. The sense of threat must be out of proportion to the event and leads to adaptive failure in what should be a stage-appropriate social engagement. Children may have a tantrum, cry, cling, or even run away as they experience the anxiety. Children with this diagnosis exhibit anxiety with peers and not solely in adult company. Some of the symptoms of social anxiety disorder and panic disorder share common transdiagnostic features, including anticipatory anxiety, panic attacks, and phobic avoidance (2).

6.2.2. Psychodynamic Factors and Conflicts

Social anxiety disorder and panic disorder share a number of central dynamics, including complicated emotional responses to separation from close attachment figures and difficulty tolerating angry feelings toward them. Clinical consensus among psychoanalytic writers indicates that patients with social anxiety disorder also have prominent conflicted exhibitionistic and grandiose fantasies and wishes (3, 4, 5, 6, 7, 8). Clarification of these dynamisms can aid in treating children and teens who suffer from social anxiety.

Symptoms of social anxiety disorder that overlap with those of panic disorder include temperamental fearfulness and terrifying perceptions of parents (9). An association has been found between social anxiety disorder and behavioral inhibition, as has been found for panic disorder (10, 11). Parents of children with behavioral inhibition were found to have higher rates of social anxiety disorder (10) and children with behavioral inhibition had higher rates of social anxiety disorder than noninhibited children (11). Temperamental fearfulness, as well as specific developmental stressors, can lead these individuals to view themselves as inadequate, incapable, or shameful and to feel easily rejected, while they often view others as ridiculing them. Persistent feelings of ineffectiveness add to a view of themselves as child-like and incompetent, while others are perceived as powerful and threatening. On the contrary, these patients are often highly critical of others when this is explored.

Children and teens with social anxiety disorder have a core sense of inadequacy and low self-esteem related to feeling incapable of being autonomous. They feel unable to act autonomously for a variety of reasons, including a sense of shame about themselves, a pervasive belief that they are too incompetent and immature to formulate responses to external situations, and worries that they will betray their close attachment figures by functioning more independently, such that potential growing autonomy could function as a terrifying threat to these relationships. Their feelings of inadequacy increase the degree of mixed emotions and conflict they experience in connection with the fantasized dangers envisioned from separation from significant others. The threat to relationships is intensified by the fantasy that powerful attachment figures are required for love, organization, and coherence. *These patients believe, often unconsciously, that socializing outside their family of origin will lead to the loss of important attachments, which results in regressive fantasies of helplessness, further increasing social anxiety, and avoidance of social situations.*

Patients develop intensely angry feelings and fantasies toward others whom they perceive as rejecting and humiliating, and in a *dynamic akin to what occurs in panic patients, they fear that their anger will pose a threat to needed relationships. Denial* and *projection of anger* are common defense mechanisms (see Box 4.5) among patients with social anxiety disorder, increasing their chances of feeling rejected and criticized. The intensity of their anger is partly fueled by feelings of helplessness and a sense of incompetence, which represent a narcissistic injury, and can be blamed on others for interfering with their development of competence. *The view of oneself as humiliated and inadequate can also serve to protect against a self-perception of being hostile and threatening, self-images that are commonly perceived to be a threat to close attachments.*

Children and adolescents with social anxiety disorder often have grandiose fantasies (i.e., out of proportion in relation to reality) that at times can be linked to conflicted sexually exhibitionistic wishes and fantasies. These fantasies may also derive from attempts to compensate for a sense of personal inadequacy.

School-aged children often learn to perform in class at the blackboard in front of the class. The child must learn in such a setting, putting aside performance anxiety and accepting instruction that can be, particularly for the self-conscious, socially phobic child, immediately interpreted as criticism. Some children who overestimate their competence or with inflated egos experience performance as a test rather than an opportunity to learn and advance their knowledge. Adolescents more often look at social performances as evaluations of aspects of their physical body displays, their attractiveness and sexiness obliterating the intent of lessons designed for learning.

Unrealistic fantasies, tinged with grandiosity, reflecting an underlying belief that one should be treated as special, often lead to disappointment in real social situations, furthering distress in response to social slights. Patients typically feel guilty when exhibitionistic and grandiose fantasies are experienced consciously, and they fear punishment, aggravating anxiety. Children and teens may avoid social situations to avoid these fantasies, likewise as a punishment for having these fantasies.

In summary, social anxiety and associated self-criticism in part represent complex compromise formations. Compromise formations are an unconscious aspect of mental life that symbolically represent a compromise between an unacceptable wish and the defense against that wish (12) (see Glossary). Social anxiety includes fears of inadequacy, humiliation and rejection, and social avoidance, which aids in averting threats to self-esteem. Social avoidance can function to maintain a regressive dependency on significant others and permit avoidance in pursuing more independent, age-appropriate relationships, which are frightening to these patients with the greater independence they imply. Social anxiety includes fears of the experience and expression of anger, and avoidance serves to avert these threats, while it may also represent an unconscious expression of contempt. Social avoidance may allow the patient to maintain a secret sense of specialness that might be challenged by responses of others. *Thus, from a psychodynamic perspective, painful shyness may be an avoidant defense against frightening aggressive, sexually exhibitionistic, and grandiose wishes, and the symptoms can also function as a punishment for these unacceptable wishes.*

6.2.3. Treatment: Transdiagnostic Techniques and Specific Adaptations

Patients with social anxiety disorder experience catastrophic fears that they are socially inadequate and will be painfully rejected and criticized. In CAPP, the therapist's approach to social phobia focuses on the emotional meanings of specific symptoms, the stressors that elicit symptoms and exacerbation, the child's developmental history, and fantasies and feelings that emerge in the transference. In this way, unconscious and warded-off fantasies and conflicts that provide the dynamic underpinnings of social phobia are identified and explored. Children and adolescents become aware that their fears derive from conflicted feelings of inadequacy, angry feelings, attachment threats, and guilt-ridden exhibitionistic and grandiose fantasies. Symptoms of social anxiety disorder improve as patients become able to identify these conflicts and as their fantasies become articulated in words, discussed and better understood, and hence detoxified.

The experience of therapy, with the nonjudgmental and empathic support of the therapist, creates an experience of tolerance of unpleasant ideas and can aid children in the development of more benign or supportive representations of themselves and others. The perceived danger of social interactions diminishes during these interventions. The CAPP therapist never directly instructs the child or adolescent to confront feared situations because this can inhibit the development of greater autonomy and can distort the transference. As psychodynamic exploration leads to reduced fears, children and adolescents naturally become more comfortable confronting situations they have been avoiding. However, mired as these patients are in taking a passive role, struggles in the transference are inevitable for children and adolescents with social phobia because their anxiety tends to rise as the therapist does not tell them what to do. When the call for guidance is not acceded to, the child may become aware of his/her anger toward the therapist. That, too, can feel untenable. The patient is caught in a quandary regarding assertiveness, which entails overriding the impending fears and acting anyway. Articulation of passive wishes in the transference and elsewhere (the wish that someone else "do" something to the person, rather than needing to take action him/herself) and articulation of the inherent dangers patients imagine they would experience in taking a more active role in their lives necessarily come to the forefront.

Addressing Conflicted Feelings and Fantasies

An important component of psychodynamic psychotherapy for children and adolescents is helping patients to become aware of, more tolerant of, and more able to express their various feelings and fantasies in words. Because of the inherent danger children and adolescents with social anxiety disorder experience about assertion of any kind, rage often feels disorganizing and threatening, and patients can find it intolerable to be angry. Nonetheless, anger frequently emerges as treatment progresses. Understanding the developmental origins of these feelings, identifying the details of related fantasies and why it seems so frightening to be angry, and the ability to safely experience this rage and disappointment in therapy allows for improved tolerance. Children with social anxiety disorder may be aware of having fantasies of grand power and being the center of attention, but often they do not connect these fantasies with the perpetuation of their social anxiety disorder. They tend to minimize the importance of these fantasies with their preoccupation with feelings of inadequacy. The therapist may identify these fantasies as they emerge in treatment and highlight their connection to the child's anxiety, even remarking that thoughts alone may not be as powerful as the child imagines them.

Countertransference

Therapists must be alert to feelings of criticism or frustration that may occur in working with children and adolescents with social anxiety disorder. Therapist frustration can be triggered by the patients' level of passivity and by their difficulty taking more autonomous steps to change their lives. This type of helplessness can engender a sense of helplessness in the therapist or alternatively the urge to pressure the child/teen into taking action, thereby shifting the internal struggle the child experiences to an interpersonal struggle, something to be avoided. Covert expression of critical feelings can lead to subtle criticisms by the therapist that can intensify the patient's feelings of inadequacy. Therapists should remain alert to their reaction to patients' sometimes contemptuous attitudes toward the therapist. Focus on the transference can help the therapist to address these conflicts. The experience of a nonjudgmental, helpful therapist who nevertheless does not direct the patient about how to specifically approach feared situations is critical in modification of negative, tormenting self and object representations. Some anxious children repeat insistent nagging and self-abnegation in the therapy in the (usually unconscious) hope of eliciting action from the therapist, which can be expected to both enrage the patient and re-enforce a sense of despised yet comfortable passivity on the part of the patient, yet also permit the patient to maintain the fantasy that the only thing that can bring about change is being "forced" by others to act. A high-stakes interpersonal struggle can emerge between child and therapist that should be articulated in words, in which the socially anxious child repeatedly unconsciously attempts to provoke the therapist into forcing him/her to act, at which point the child would be likely to refuse, often triumphantly. Rather than falling into the trap of acting out the dictatorial side of this schematized relationship, the therapist should verbally place the interpersonal conundrum before the child: demonstrating that nothing the therapist can "do" in this situation (try to force the child to act, versus not doing so) would feel comfortable to the child. Discussions such as this can help the child to both understand and own both sides of the conflict he or she faces. Interpersonal problems of this kind have been called "masochistic provocation."

6.2.4. Cases: Fifteen-Year-Old John and Eighteen-Year-Old Brian

John, a 15-year-old sophomore in high school, diagnosed with social anxiety disorder, always felt his strong points were in History and English, using these as markers of his positive social identity. However, he did not trust his math skills. He linked these anxieties to his mediocre sports ability. He shrank from performing, especially in those arenas, and hid in the last rows of his classes or frequently missed gym class when team sports were scheduled. When asked to perform, he mumbled, chalked the board lightly and tentatively, and flushed. Noticing his timidity in such positions, teachers learned to avoid calling on him.

Eighteen-year-old Brian, by contrast, offered a grand and overblown pride in his grasp of school subjects, but when the acknowledgement he imagined was not forthcoming, he shrank back and resisted future situations in which he might have to perform. He had not yet recognized that his performance was unconsciously designed to be an aggressive assault on his classmates and teachers, angrily seeking to "knock 'em dead" in his fantasies, rather than to inform or entertain them. Somehow these fantasies managed to be communicated to others without his being aware of it. These early experiences continued to plague Brian's adaptive engagement in life, and he was diagnosed at age 18 as having social anxiety disorder.

These two examples show that social anxiety disorder can manifest clinically in a number of ways, depending on the individual defense mechanisms the child/teen adopts.

References

1. American Psychiatric Association. (2013). *Diagnostic and statistical manual of mental disorders* (5th ed.). Washington, DC: American Psychiatric Press.
2. American Psychiatric Association. (2000). *Diagnostic and statistical manual of mental disorders* (4th ed., text revision). Washington, DC: American Psychiatric Press.
3. Fenichel, O. (1945). *The psychoanalytic theory of neurosis.* New York, NY: W. W. Norton.
4. Gabbard, G. O. (2000). *Psychodynamic psychiatry in clinical practice* (3rd ed.). Washington, DC: American Psychiatric Press.
5. Gabbard, G. O. (1992). Psychodynamics of panic disorder and social phobia. *Bulletin of the Menninger Clinic, 56* (2, Suppl. A), A3–A13.
6. Kaplan, D. M. (1972). On shyness. *International Journal of Psychoanalysis, 53,* 439–454.
7. Zerbe, K. J. (1994). Uncharted waters: Psychodynamic considerations in the diagnosis and treatment of social phobia. *Bulletin of the Menninger Clinic, 58*(2, Suppl. A), A3–20.
8. Lipsitz, J. D., & Marshall, R. D. (2001). Alternative psychotherapy approaches for social anxiety disorder. *Psychiatric Clinics of North America, 24,* 817–829.
9. Arrindell, W. A., Emmelkamp, P. M. G., Monsma, A., & Brilman, E. (1983). The role of perceived parental rearing practices in the aetiology of phobic disorder: A controlled study. *British Journal of Psychiatry, 143,* 183–187.
10. Rosenbaum, J. F., Biederman, J., Hirshfeld, D. R., Bolduc, E. A., Faraone, S. J., Kagan, J., . . . Reznick, J. S. (1991). Further evidence of an association between behavioral inhibition and anxiety disorders: Results from a family study of children from a non-clinical sample. *Journal of Psychiatric Research, 25,* 49–65.
11. Biederman, J., Hirshfeld-Becker, D. R., Rosenbaum, J. F., Hérot, C., Friedman, D., Snidman, . . . Faraone, S. V. (2001). Further evidence of association between behavioral inhibition and social anxiety in children. *American Journal of Psychiatry, 158*(10), 1673–1679.
12. Freud, S. (1955). *Studies in hysteria* (Standard ed. 2). London, UK: Hogarth Press (Originally published in 1893/1895).

6.3. Separation Anxiety Disorder With Case Vignette

6.3.1. Symptoms, Signs, and Diagnostic Considerations

The core feature of separation anxiety disorder (SAD) is excessive and developmentally inappropriate anxiety or distress when faced with actual or anticipated separation from major attachment figures. As defined in DSM-5 (1), symptoms of SAD include excessive distress when facing or anticipating separation from home or attachment figures as well as persistent worries about permanently losing or being abandoned by attachments or of potential harm that may befall them during separations (such as the person falling ill, getting into an accident, or dying). Children and teens with SAD may be afraid to be alone or without a parent/attachment figure close at hand and may avoid developmentally normative tasks such as going to school, being outside of the home in general, sleeping in bed alone, or sleeping away from home because of separation fears. If persistent, these inhibitions lead to increasing non-normative development, with an accumulation of failures to attain culturally-expected norms. Physical symptoms and somatic complaints are commonly associated with separation concerns and may include headaches, stomachaches, nausea, vomiting, or panic-like symptoms of autonomic hyperarousal. Among children with SAD, school refusal is common (2). Yet, school refusal can be associated with a variety of childhood mood and anxiety disorders (3); these are distinguishable from SAD in terms of primary symptomatic preoccupation (4).

Current DSM criteria require that SAD symptoms cause clinically significant distress or functional impairment and have a minimum duration of four weeks in children and adolescents. SAD has historically been considered a disorder of infancy, childhood, or adolescence, with DSM-IV (5) criteria requiring onset before age 18, a requirement that was lifted in DSM-5.

SAD is a common childhood anxiety disorder (6, 7, 8). Age of first onset is estimated at seven to nine years (9, 10, 11), which is earlier than the age of onset for other DSM anxiety disorders in childhood (10). Higher rates of childhood SAD have been observed in girls (12, 13, 14, 15), who may be twice as likely as boys to experience SAD (11, 12).

Uncommonly in the domain of anxiety disorders, most cases of SAD appear to go undetected, and like other anxiety disorders, undertreatment is the norm. National Comorbidity Survey Replication data indicate that only 21.8% of individuals meeting criteria for childhood SAD received treatment during childhood; among those who received childhood treatment, only 24.3% reported that SAD was a focus of treatment (9), a troubling omission. Aspects of the symptomatology of SAD can become reinforced by anxious families and can be ego syntonic, which may further contribute to inadequate therapeutic interventions (16).

It has now been convincingly demonstrated that childhood SAD is a potent precursor, or risk factor, for subsequent development of other anxiety and mood disorders in later childhood and adulthood. Solid data from numerous sources now exist that demonstrate this (17, 18). For this reason, among others, treatment of SAD in childhood is crucial.

6.3.2. Psychodynamic Factors and Conflicts

Children and teens with SAD struggle to feel age-competent because of their need to keep parents closer than what is culturally considered age-normative. They have difficulty feeling independent or doing more independent things (depending on their stage of development, this might be sleeping through the night, going to school without mother, or having a sleepover), which invariably leads to anxiety and a sense of personal incompetence. Core underlying fantasies tend to involve being abandoned—or abandoning—their close attachment figures (usually parents), often experienced as the world being dangerous when they are not with these caretakers. This preoccupation speaks to these children's underlying discomfort with the safety and the durability of their attachments as well as discomfort with any ambivalence they may be feeling within those relationships. Some of these children do not feel "complete" as people without the presence of their separation attachment figure. No matter what the quality of the relationship with the therapist has been before the termination phase of CAPP, it is invariable that for these children that make fears of separation will necessarily emerge in the transference, making termination a key time to address these conflicts and set of feelings.

6.3.3. Treatment: Transdiagnostic Techniques and Specific Adaptations

Specific therapeutic techniques in CAPP that focus on SAD revolve around the therapist very carefully tracking the child's responses to the new attachment relationship with the therapist as it evolves. Inserting excessive references to the relationship with the therapist early in treatment is usually distracting to children. Unless the child/teen is having ambivalence or difficulty coming to the sessions, this information should be kept in mind by the therapist in order to make links later as treatment unfolds between what is happening in the relationship in the room and its connections to other difficulties with separation and attachment in the patient's life. The therapist should openly take note of the child's responses to missed appointments or variations in schedule during the treatment as a way of bringing separation and any ambivalence about autonomy into the verbal discussion in the room. The transference relationship requires articulation and exploration, even if there appear to be no problems and the patient is feeling better. Specific things to explore might be: Why does the child think he/she is feeling better? What might have calmed the child down? The therapist is seeking as accurate a way as possible to verbally capture the child's relationship to the therapist. CAPP treatment of SAD uses the transference as an emotionally vibrant paradigm for understanding and altering separation fears. Intensity (twice weekly) and brevity (12 weeks) are key aspects of CAPP, and the emotional significance of termination is a central topic at minimum of the final third of treatment.

6.3.4. Case: Eight-Year-Old Marissa

Marissa was eight years old when she entered therapy because her mother noted that she was having trouble making friends in her new school. Marissa had switched schools for third grade because her mother thought Marissa was feeling put off at the school she attended for first and second grade, which was a religious school of a different denomination than Marissa's family. Marissa told her mother she was the only child of her faith in her whole grade, and as a result, she felt uncomfortable during the school's mandatory daily chapels and religion classes. Marissa's mother thought Marissa's complaints justified the school change (to a nondenominational school) and also adequately explained the fact that Marissa had made no friends at school. "Everyone in the class has country houses and we don't," Mrs. X told the therapist when they met. "It really didn't occur to me that Marissa was having basic problems making friends, or being away from me."

Marissa's mother's lack of awareness about Marissa's separation anxiety symptoms is typical of parents of children with SAD. The disorder is often normalized and accepted for a very long time before treatment is sought.

Marissa cried every morning before she went to the new school. It emerged that this pattern was a long-established one from her mornings in the old school. In the morning, she frequently vomited her breakfast and begged to stay home. Her mother acceded to her wishes some of the time, which she had done to an even greater extent in the old school.

In therapy, Marissa was initially somewhat shy, but it was noteworthy that her mother offered to stay in the room with her and the therapist long after Marissa wanted to "just come in and play." Marissa played with the family dolls in sessions, constructing elaborate stories about nervous mothers and daughters, with mothers alternating between being calm and rational, encouraging the girls to go out and make new friends, and being extremely worried about every little thing the children did, asking very bothersome questions about every word the girls said to other children and teachers, as though it was hard for the mothers to be separate from the children. It was gradually through the play that Marissa was able to discuss her sense of her own mother's difficulty separating from her, and the therapist made a link between the anxious mothers and Marissa's mother, particularly as they had observed in the waiting room and in her therapy.

References

1. American Psychiatric Association. (2013). *Diagnostic and statistical manual of mental disorders* (5th ed.). Washington, DC: American Psychiatric Press.
2. Eisen, A. R., & Schaefer, C. E. (2008). *Separation anxiety in children and adolescents: An individualized approach to assessment and treatment.* Princeton, NJ: Recording for the Blind & Dyslexic.
3. Kearney, C. A. (2007). Forms and functions of school refusal behavior in youth: An empirical analysis of absenteeism severity. *Journal of Child Psychology and Psychiatry, 48*(1):53–61.
4. Cyranowski, J. M., Shear, M. K., Rucci, P., Fagiolini, A., Frank, E., Grochocinski, V. J., . . . Cassano, G. (2002). Adult separation anxiety: Psychometric properties of a new structured clinical interview. *Journal of Psychiatric Research, 36*(2):77–86.
5. American Psychiatric Association. (1994). *Diagnostic criteria from diagnostic and statistical manual of mental disorders* (4th ed.). Washington, DC: American Psychiatric Press.
6. Compton, S. N., Nelson, A. H., & March, J. S. (2000). Social phobia and separation anxiety symptoms in community and clinical samples of children and adolescents. *Journal of the American Academy of Child and Adolescent Psychiatry, 39*(8), 1040–1046.

7. Allen, J. L., Rapee, R. M., & Sandberg, S. (2008). Severe life events and chronic adversities as antecedents to anxiety in children: A matched control study. *Journal of Abnormal Child Psychology*, *36*(7): 1047–1056.

8. Keller, M. B., Lavori, P. W., Wunder, J., Beardslee, W. R., Schwartz, C. E., & Roth, J. (1992). Chronic course of anxiety disorders in children and adolescents. *Journal of the American Academy of Child and Adolescent Psychiatry*, *31*(4), 595–599.

9. Shear, K., Jin, R., Ruscio, A. M., Walters, E. E., & Kessler, R. C. (2006). Prevalence and correlates of estimated DSM-IV child and adult separation anxiety disorder in the National Comorbidity Survey Replication. *American Journal of Psychiatry*, *163*(6), 1074–1083.

10. Bacow, T. L., Pincus, D. B., Ehrenreich, J. T., & Brody, L. R. (2009). The metacognitions questionnaire for children: Development and validation in a clinical sample of children and adolescents with anxiety disorders. *Journal of Anxiety Disorders*, *23*(6), 727–736.

11. Foley, D. L., Rowe, R., Maes, H., Silberg, J., Eaves, L., & Pickles, A. (2008). The relationship between separation anxiety and impairment. *Journal of Anxiety Disorders*, *22*(4), 635–641.

12. Bowen, R. C., Offord, D. R., Boyle, M. H. (1990). The prevalence of overanxious disorder and separation anxiety disorder: Results from the Ontario Child Health Study. *Journal of the American Academy of Child and Adolescent Psychiatry*, *29*(5), 753–758.

13. Anderson, J. C., Williams, S., McGee, R., & Silva, P. A. (1987). DSM-III disorders in preadolescent children: Prevalence in a large sample from the general population. *Archives of General Psychiatry*, *44*(1), 69–76.

14. Lewinsohn, P. M., Hops, H., Roberts, R. E., Seeley, J. R., & Andrews, J. A. (1993). Adolescent psychopathology. I. Prevalence and incidence of depression and other DSM-III-R disorders in high school students. *Journal of Abnormal Psychology*, *102*(1), 133–144.

15. Lewinsohn, P. M., Holm-Denoma, J. M., Small, J. W., Seeley, J. R., & Joiner, T. E. (2008). Separation anxiety disorder in childhood as a risk factor for future mental illness. *Journal of the American Academy of Child and Adolescent Psychiatry*, *47*(5):548–555.

16. Milrod, B., Markowitz, J. C., Gerber, A. J., Cyranowski, J., Altemus, M., Shapiro, T., . . . Glatt, C. (2014). Childhood separation anxiety and the pathogenesis and treatment of adult anxiety. *American Journal of Psychiatry*, *171*(1), 34–43.

17. Kossowsky, J., Pfaltz, M. C., Schneider, S., Taeymans, J., Locher, C., & Gaab, J. (2013). The separation anxiety hypothesis of panic disorder revisited: A meta-analysis. *American Journal of Psychiatry*, *170*, 768–781.

18. Silove, D., Alonso, J., Bromet, E., Gruber, M., Sampson, N., Scott, K., . . . Kessler, R. C. (2015). Pediatric-onset and adult-onset separation anxiety disorder across countries in the World Mental Health Survey. *American Journal of Psychiatry*, *172*(7), 647–656.

6.4. Panic Disorder With Case Vignette

6.4.1. Symptoms, Signs, and Diagnostic Considerations

Panic disorder is characterized by recurrent panic attacks that seem to the child to emerge from nowhere specifically. Panic attacks themselves are characterized by at least four of nine autonomic symptoms of sympathomimetic rush (1), some of which may be more cognitive (i.e., the sense of derealization or depersonalization) rather than purely physical sensations. Panic attacks tend to last 10 to 15 minutes and gradually subside. While panic attacks can occur with a very wide range of psychiatric disorders, panic disorder is only diagnosed if kids are preoccupied or worried about the attacks or have a sense that something is wrong with them because of them. Children and teens with panic disorder tend to worry that they will get future attacks. These worries often limit what they feel comfortable doing. Panic disorder can occur with or without agoraphobia, and both panic attacks and agoraphobia can accompany mood and anxiety disorders.

6.4.2. Psychodynamic Factors and Conflicts

Through the exploration of the very specific circumstances and feelings accompanying anxiety and panic onset, the therapist and the child/teen are able to develop an increasing understanding of the, at least partially, unconscious conflicts central to panic and anxiety. Themes that emerge over time in therapy often involve conflicts about separation, anger toward close attachment figures, mixed feelings about sexuality, and guilt. The therapist helps the child/teen to elucidate how these conflicts lead to anxiety symptoms. These conflicts will now be described in greater depth.

Conflicts About Separation and Autonomy

Worries about and even fantasies surrounding separation and autonomy are often areas of conflict for severely anxious, panicking patients. There is indirect support for this clinical finding in the literature from several epidemiological sources (2, 3). Weissman et al. (4), in the Yale Family Study, found that the presence of panic disorder in parents conferred more than a threefold risk for separation anxiety disorder in their offspring between the ages of six and 17. Rosenbaum et al. (5) found that 84.6% of offspring of parents with panic disorder and agoraphobia demonstrated behavioral inhibition (BI) at significantly greater frequency than a comparison group of children of probands with other psychiatric disorders. This risk may reflect genetic, psychological vulnerabilities, or both. Recent twin studies by Eley et al. point toward a definitive role of epigenetic, or environmental, factors in development of anxiety (6).

Children and teens commonly report that life events preceding panic attack onset involve real or fantasized loss or separation, often from people about whom they feel ambivalent. In our clinical experience with adults with panic disorder, we have noted that dealing with loss and separation, whether in reality or symbolically, is an important aspect of panic onset and persistence. We found that 73% of adult patients with primary DSM-IV panic disorder presenting to a clinical trial of psychotherapy had panic onset within 6 weeks of experiencing an interpersonal loss event, defined as death of a close attachment figure, breakup of a serious relationship or divorce, or miscarriage/abortion (7). Thoughts accompanying panic attacks typically involve fear of being alone and unable to care for oneself. Adults and children with PD both feel incompetent and as if they cannot survive alone, or at the developmental level expected of them. A phobic companion (often a parent) is frequently felt to be necessary to protect against this and other dangers, which is consistent with the well-known association between panic disorder and agoraphobia (8, 9, 10, 11).

A psychodynamic psychotherapy of any anxiety disorder involving prominent panic attacks must therefore investigate the child's intense fears of separation and his/her sense of not being able to function when alone as would be appropriate to his/her present developmental stage. These fears have their origins in conflictual events from earlier in childhood and are necessarily connected to ongoing interpersonal difficulties. Earlier temperamental and emotional precursors, as described by Busch et al. (12) and Shear et al. (13), set the stage for a separation-individuation process riddled with disappointments and conflicts and for future (later childhood and teenage) difficulties with modulation of anxiety and interpersonal intimacy, as are common for patients with attachment dysregulation.

These issues will necessarily arise in the child's developing relationship with the therapist. For example, children and teens with panic disorder fear becoming "overly dependent" on their therapists, as they have felt with other important people in their lives, most notably with parents. This can be manifested in the therapeutic situation by the teenager's frequently finding reasons to miss sessions, or in the other extreme, to come very early and to wait for hours before sessions. For some children and teens, these fears will make it difficult for them to become engaged in psychotherapy. In CAPP, it is important to pay attention to what extent parents may play an active role in thwarting the child's engagement in therapy because of the (often unconscious) psychological meanings the child's symptom has for them, or how the symptoms affect the child's dependence on them. Other children with panic disorder become quite dependent on the therapist and respond with mounting terror or intense sadness or anger to changes in meeting times, therapist vacations, and looming termination. The therapeutic setting, by its very nature, provides many natural inroads for the exploration and re-emergence of this important set of conflicts.

Conflicts Over Anger

Clinical observations suggest that patients with panic disorder have intense difficulties tolerating and modulating their angry feelings and thoughts (12, 13). Fear of anger, and the conscious and unconscious vindictive fantasies that go along with this feeling, are frequent precipitants of panic attacks. The therapist must approach the child in a manner that will facilitate exploration of angry feelings and the accompanying fantasies that are perceived as dangerous. A nonjudgmental stance is important because these children and teens often need for a variety of reasons to see themselves as "not angry." Helping the child become aware of at least partially unconscious anger and to begin to understand what he/she is afraid of is an important tool in panic resolution. Helping children and teens distinguish fantasies from realistic concerns and helping them handle anger in an effective way are also crucial parts of CAPP.

The way in which a child's family manages anger can be informative. Familial difficulties with the management of rage or hostility can manifest in overt family acrimony and violence. It is not uncommon for parental anxiety to be expressed as rage toward the child/teen. For example, parents who are consumed with fears about their teens' well-being and safety at times when they break rules, such as when they come home late after curfew, may express their fears as rage toward the teen when they are reunited. The teenager's unconscious childhood understanding of the often-unstated significance of parents' anxiety symptoms, such as fears that the teen will be attacked if he/she is out late, becomes incorporated into fantasies about the meaning of the expression of his/her own rage and anxiety symptoms.

Conflicts about anger can make it difficult for children and teens with panic attacks to discuss their feelings and fantasies directly in treatment. For example, some children have observed uncontrollable anger in their parents and are frightened that they will be harmed. Understandably, these fears translate to the current psychotherapeutic relationship and can contribute to reticence about expressing or acknowledging anger. These factors must be incorporated into the therapist's understanding of the meaning of the child's panic attacks and in the timing and structure of therapeutic interventions.

Common fantasies are that rage or its expression will result in abandonment by the people on whom the child most depends. Unconscious homicidal fantasies conflicting with loving feelings can be central in children's difficulty in both feeling close and being able to separate in a normative way. *These fears are not necessarily connected to actual experiences but can nonetheless represent compelling, organizing fantasies.*

Inhibitions in discussing these topics in psychotherapy can take place in relationship to the child's fear of acknowledging angry feelings toward the therapist, who necessarily serves as a model for the patient's important, conflicted relationships.

Conflicts About Sexual Excitement

Although panic attacks often occur in the setting of conflicted hostility, for some patients, particularly teenagers who struggle with their relatively newly sexual bodies and roles, the attacks also can take on a significance of their own, beyond the commonly experienced, manifest panic thoughts of being ill and dying or becoming "crazy." For some teenagers, panic episodes themselves are inherently frightening and arousing and can be closely tied to sadomasochistic sexual fantasies and conflicts. These teens frequently present complaining about their panic attacks but may be surprisingly reluctant to be rid of them. Patients say that without the constant anxiety with which they have been living, life would seem "boring" (14) and that the attacks provide excitement, content ["it's part of who I am and it defines me"], and for some, a distraction from more disturbing (e.g., violent and sexual) thoughts and fantasies.

Panic attacks, like any symptom, may take on various intrapsychic meanings for patients and central meanings may shift over time. It is not until these secondary dynamic reinforcers of the symptoms are also grasped, and alternative methods are found for the patient to cope with these conflicts, that the symptoms can be successfully relinquished. In the therapeutic setting, these dynamics may emerge in arousing struggles, often engineered unconsciously by the teenage patient with the therapist.

6.4.3. Treatment: Transdiagnostic Techniques and Specific Adaptations

The initial evaluation of the child or teen with panic disorder or other severe anxiety disorders that feature prominent panic attacks includes an assessment of both panic attacks and associated anxiety symptoms that occur during and around the attacks. The psychodynamically oriented clinician explores the child's personality characteristics (i.e., how the child tends to respond to particular stressors over time, along with chronic views of himself/herself and others that form a backdrop to life history, level of functioning, and perception of significant relationships). The child or teen's ability to express himself/herself in words will constitute an important consideration for the CAPP therapist in terms of types of interventions that will be necessary early on in psychotherapy in order to make the treatment understandable to the child. In the evaluation, attention should be paid to topics that are uncomfortable, or are defended, which is manifested by the child/teen finding them difficult to discuss or rapidly changing the subject.

The following guidelines cover areas that are important in panic and anxiety assessment. However, these guidelines should not be adhered to rigidly.

1. Assessment of Panic Attacks and Physiological Symptoms of Anxiety
   - Symptoms as per DSM-5
   - Very careful delineation of situations preceding panic onset: circumstances, feelings, and stressors, such as losses, changes in location, or alteration in level of responsibilities or relationships with significant others
   - Description of prior panic episodes or episodes of physical anxiety symptoms with associated symptoms, thoughts, feelings, and circumstances of onset; this is often tracked by children and teens as times in which they were "sick," as the experience of panic can feel as though it is a physical illness
2. Developmental History
   - Perception of parents and family life with attention focused on the way in which anger, anxiety, physical illness, and other emotional topics are managed in the family; a history of early losses and separations is crucial
   - Earlier childhood anxiety symptoms: school phobias, shyness, childhood fears and worries since infancy
   - Adolescence (if applicable): dependence/autonomy conflicts, relationships, struggles around control, anxiety management; the way in which anger, separation, and sexuality are handled
3. Assessment of the Child/Teen's Ease of Adaptation to a Psychodynamic Approach
   - Assessment of the ability to think psychologically, to describe relationships to others, to make dynamic connections, to put feelings into words, and to maintain curiosity about one's motivation and role in one's difficulties

Psychodynamic psychotherapy works well even in psychologically unsophisticated patients, but the therapist may need to explain why he/she is saying what he/she says in greater depth for some children.

Motivation is often very high in psychotherapy for children and teens with panic and anxiety disorders when they begin a new treatment because they experience such a high degree of distress about their symptoms that they are often ready to work seriously in psychotherapy. The therapist should actively and verbally note dynamic themes that emerge during the assessment to the child as a part of the evaluation process in order to assess his/her comfort and ability to make connections to psychological meanings of the panic attacks. These factors will form a backdrop to the psychotherapeutic approach at the outset of treatment that will shape elements of the intervention itself.

6.4.4. Case: Eighteen-Year-Old William

William, an 18-year-old high school senior who had multiple daily panic episodes, kept himself close to a panic state at all times by drinking quarts of strong coffee. When this was explored in psychotherapy, William said that he "loved" the feeling of being so "wound up" that he was always close to a state of panic. "It's exciting," he said.

William became extremely anxious at times when he felt passive, "unmanly," or vulnerable. His early childhood history of having been sexually seduced by his mother was closely connected with his fear of being passive. Staying close to a panicky, ultra-alert state served to protect him from disturbing passive longings that were unconsciously represented by his panic attacks themselves.

With his therapist, William frequently initiated struggles about who was in charge, with the conscious feeling that he always wanted to be, even though he often begged "to be ordered" to do things, such as his homework. It was initially hard for him to acknowledge that he did this, but as is often the case, the process that he underwent with others (mother, teachers) was easier for him to explore when it emerged in the transference. This example came from the second month of his psychotherapy.

> WILLIAM: Tell me what to talk about. I'm not going to talk about anything till you tell me what to say. I might talk about things that are unimportant, and waste my time here.
>
> THERAPIST: It sounds like you want me to order you around so much that you won't even talk without my prior approval.
>
> WILLIAM: Well, I don't know what's important. You do. You just don't want to tell me.
>
> THERAPIST: At the moment, what seems clear is that you feel that I'm neglecting you, depriving you of my knowledge, and that you're angry at me. But it does seem that this whole process, of being in a struggle with me, happens over and over.
>
> WILLIAM: I know. (He grins and giggles.)
>
> THERAPIST: It seems like there's something a little fun about being in a fight with me.

It gradually became clear that William found these struggles intensely exciting. He brought them about repeatedly, grinned and became physically jittery when they occurred.

Teasing out these exciting issues in the treatment became important in this teenager's relinquishing his panic symptoms.

References

1. American Psychiatric Association. (2013). *Diagnostic and statistical manual of mental disorders* (5th ed.). Washington, DC: American Psychiatric Press.
2. Kossowsky, J., Pfaltz, M. C., Schneider, S., Taeymans, J., Locher, C., & Gaab, J. (2013). The separation anxiety hypothesis of panic disorder revisited: a meta-analysis. *American Journal of Psychiatry, 170*(7), 768–781.
3. Silove, D., Alonso, J., Bromet, E., Gruber, M., Sampson, N., Scott, K., . . . Kessler, R. C. (2015). Pediatric-onset and adult-onset separation anxiety disorder across countries in the World Mental Health Survey. *American Journal of Psychiatry, 172*(7), 647–656.
4. Weissman, M. M., Leckman, J. F., & Merikengas, K. R. (1984). Depression and anxiety disorders in parents and children: Results from the Yale Family Study. *Archives of General Psychiatry, 41*, 845–852.
5. Rosenbaum, J. F., Biederman, J., Gersten, M., Hirshfeld, D. R., Meminger, S. R., Herman, J. B., . . . Snidman, M. (1988). Behavioral inhibition in children of parents with panic disorder and agoraphobia: A controlled study. *Archives of General Psychiatry, 45*(5), 463–470.
6. Eley, T. C., McAdams, T. A., Rijsdijk, F. V., Lichtenstein, P., Narusyte, J., Reiss, D., . . . Neiderhiser, J. M. (2015). The intergenerational transmission of anxiety: A children-of-twins study. *American Journal of Psychiatry, 172*(7), 630–637.
7. Klass, E. T., Milrod, B., Leon, A. C., Kay, S. J, Schwalberg, M., Li, C., & Markowitz, J. C. (2009). Does interpersonal loss preceding panic disorder onset moderate response to psychotherapy? An exploratory study. *Journal of Clinical Psychiatry, 70*(3), 406–411.
8. Freud, S. (1895). On the grounds for detaching a particular syndrome from neurasthenia under the description "anxiety neurosis" (Standard ed. 3, pp. 85–115). London, UK: Hogarth Press.
9. Freud, S. (1926). Inhibitions, symptoms and anxiety (Standard ed. 20, pp. 75–126). London, UK: Hogarth Press.
10. Klein, D. F., & Gorman, J. M. (1987). A model of panic and agoraphobic development. *Acta Psychiatrica Scandinavia Supplement, 335*, 87–95.
11. American Psychiatric Association. (2013). *Diagnostic criteria from diagnostic and statistical manual of mental disorders* (5th ed.). Washington, DC: American Psychiatric Press.
12. Busch, F. N., Cooper, A. M., Klerman, G. L., Penzer, R. J., Shapiro, T., & Shear, K. M. (1991). Neurophysiological, cognitive-behavioral, on psychoanalytic approaches to panic disorder: Toward an integration. *Psychoanalytic Inquiry, 11*(3), 316–332.
13. Shear, M. K., Cooper, A. M., Klerman, G. L., Busch, F. N., & Shapiro, T. (1993). A psychodynamic model of panic disorder. *American Journal of Psychiatry, 150*(6): 859–866.
14. Milrod, B. (2007). Emptiness in agoraphobia patients. *Journal of the American Psychoanalytic Association, 55*(3), 1007–1026.

6.5. Agoraphobia and Phobic Avoidance With Case Vignette

6.5.1. Symptoms, Signs, and Diagnostic Considerations

Agoraphobia is characterized by marked fear or anxiety about two or more of the following: public transportation, open spaces, enclosed spaces, crowds, or simply being outside the home. The agoraphobic child avoids situations in which he/she feels that escape is difficult for fear of having a panic attack or incontinence. The fear is out of proportion to the danger in reality and is sometimes ameliorated by having a trusted companion (1) with him/her.

The term *agoraphobia* comes from Greek and is translated as "fear of the market-place" or of open spaces from which escape would be difficult. The idea of agoraphobia has been expanded to include difficulty going to less familiar places; patients often draw magical boundaries of "safe" versus "dangerous" places. Agoraphobia is a grand avoidance technique, unconsciously designed by the patient to cling to home and the familiar. It is, when so translated, an extreme variant of separation anxiety that keeps the child or adolescent close to the safe base from which exploration has often been impossible and therefore has the developmental burden of a fright response and regression away from autonomy-seeking and exploration. Phenomenologically, agoraphobia can be a close cousin of school avoidance or school phobia (2). The task of childhood and adolescent development of increasing comfort with increasing degrees of autonomy and the ability to explore the surroundings has been abandoned in these children and adolescents for the, necessarily magical, safety of home. In this instance, we can see variant forms of such avoidance as development of somatic symptoms, nausea in the morning, appetite loss, or dawdling and sleeping in before school.

The natural history of agoraphobia may begin with the gradual withdrawal from the larger world because of anxiety that begins often in a *displaced avoidance of external events.* The fantasized "safety" of home is often a fiction because family conflict is significant for most of these patients. Alternatively, symptoms may start with generalizing a bullying event or a rejection by peers outside the home that registers in poor self-esteem, or with phobic transformation of a thing or place or animal encountered outside the home that in itself should not elicit anxiety. The cat- or dog-phobic child may by chance see a dog in his/her apartment building elevator or on the lawn and then withdraw to the closed door with the anticipation of danger afoot anywhere outside the refuge. The true agoraphobic child inhabits an alternate, magical fantasy world, in which places and spaces are either magically dangerous, and hence avoided, or magically labeled as "safe," which also constitutes a denial of realistic dangers that can occur anywhere. Severe agoraphobia involves a disturbance in the child's relationship to reality on some level, and in this way treatment must address the child's fragile and at times evanescent bond to reality, and aspects of the child's own identity (3). The events that lead to agoraphobia may have a linear or broken story line, but that story becomes the psychological underpinning of the avoidance and the contingency chain in a behavioral sense. *Ideas of magical safety and danger are central to unraveling the meaning of any given agoraphobic set of symptoms. Disturbances in identity formation and uncertainty regarding public presentation often enhance the radical avoidance that constitutes agoraphobia.*

The extremity of the defensive withdrawal is often related to panic attacks and extreme anxiety, which drive the avoidance to a fantasized safety in the home or to a single room where the *aura of safety* and *fantasy* or *memory* of a *protective buffering mother* or other attachment figure can be trusted to cushion the anxiety and secure the anxious child.

The agoraphobic child may have one or few companions who can be trusted to accompany him/her outside the home. That individual usually has a complex role in the person's life. Most often it is an ambivalently held representative of a safe base, but also it is someone against whom hostility has to be contained (1). Historically, the agoraphobic child has often experienced the threat of abandonment in some cases and frank abuse in others. The phobic companion is often kept in sight so that the child's feared but displaced aggressive fantasies projected toward the companion can be repeatedly demonstrated not to be real, in the organizing aggressive fantasies hence demonstrated to be false. This need to have the ambivalently-held phobic companion close is yet another demonstration of the child's fragile relationship to reality. The expression of killing someone in thought applies. An anxious child thought of as passive and worried can be extremely controlling at home, can disrupt family plans, spoil outings, and arouse his/her parents' anger and elicits threats. These acts of impatience are interpreted by the vulnerable child as aggressive, rejecting, and dangerous to safety for fear of abandonment or reprisal. They underscore these children's fear of their own assertiveness and anger. Thus the loved, and at the same time hated, companion must be watched closely, and *clinging often emerges as a compromise expression of rage and attachment* (ambivalent or "dysregulated" attachments).

Behavioral techniques are often resorted to in treatment of children with agoraphobia, using exposure or gradual re-entry to the external environment. If such approaches are not successful, the agoraphobic child may become further entrenched in hopelessness, guilt, and rage at the behavioral therapist that can encompass a myriad of conflicts, including that so many individuals, and some dear to him/her, have been putting so much effort into disengaging him/her from the home. The approach in dynamic therapy that respects these children's inner story and reasons for fear opens the possibilities for gradual disengagement that comes from the child him/herself, rather than via external mandates, from the confining fantasied safety while gradually opening up new and exciting opportunities for enjoyment of stage-related social experiences. This involves deeper exploration of inner experiences and conflicted relationships.

6.5.2. Psychodynamic Factors and Conflicts

Phobic behaviors require careful differentiation from the pool of anxiety disorders. Phobic objects emerge from defensive mechanisms and experiential displacements from fearful encounters onto inappropriate substitutes (a mislabeling of dangers). Common phobias in the young include dogs and birthday parties and, later, schools or locales where one expects anxiety provocation to arise. Agoraphobia can be an extension of early separation fears and an extension of avoidance as a style that can blur into more global magical thinking and fearfulness. The phobic companion is but another version of intensified dynamisms of separation anxiety.

It is essential to explore the *secondary gain in the family around the phobia*. For example, "Mommy and Daddy stop fighting when I'm scared," or "I get to take special walks with Mommy." If huge reinforcements of the phobia occur by the family, the therapist may need to schedule a family meeting to explicitly address the family's active role in the perpetuation of the phobia.

6.5.3. Treatment: Transdiagnostic Techniques and Specific Adaptations

The central approach to handling phobic avoidance in a short-term psychodynamic treatment is to focus on the *magical quality of the phobia operating as though fantasies and fears have become real in the external world.* In other words, to maintain the belief that is central to the phobia's persistence, the child must somehow convince himself/herself that the world is artificially divided between magically "safe" places and magically "dangerous" places. This involves constructing magical "danger" haloes as well as magical "safe" ones, on which less focus is often consciously placed. *Exploration of this overarching fantasy intrusion/magical organization of the world must be actively explored in the following manner:*

1. It is important that the child fully describe the detailed fabric of the magical fantasy underlying the phobia: Which specific places are safe? Which places are dangerous? Why are they dangerous in fantasy? *The therapist must build a clear picture in his/her mind of what the child's fantasy is before trying to articulate underlying reasons or suggest understandings.* The therapist needs to be explicit about the magical, fantasy nature of these dangers throughout the discussion. The therapist clarifies that the dangers are not "real" or truly dangerous in the real world but that *they represent important emotional dangers in some way that we will discover together.* Anxious children are almost always quite clear that their phobias do not represent reality, but this reassurance from the therapist serves as a support of reality, providing enough short-term relief of anxiety to permit further exploration. The focus is on identifying affectively driven, unconscious fantasies as the source of the perceived danger with the purpose of finding and labeling what in fact *is* dangerous. The central idea here is that there is a danger, in fact an *internal one,* but that it is *being misperceived and therefore mislabeled as coming from someplace outside of the realm of the child's own emotional experience.*

2. What does the child see as the origin of, and perhaps authority for, these ideas about safety and danger? The connections between the child's fantasies and the origins about danger, such as scary movies that connect to underlying fantasies, must be specifically delineated. Sometimes these ideas connect with parents and siblings and can be overt (e.g., "my older brother told me") or unspoken ("my mother never goes past the haunted house"). It can also be helpful to ask the child to think about, "What's the worst that can happen?"

3. When did the child start to believe these phobic things? Was it just "always" like this? Was it at a particular developmental moment (e.g., birth of sibling, starting at a new school), or did it start after a traumatic event (I was stuck in the elevator)? If the onset is traumatic, as in the elevator example—what was so frightening about the experience itself? If the phobia carries a symbolic link to a loss or sad event (e.g., "after Barney the dog died, I can never be alone in the dark"), the therapist must explore and articulate emotional links between the loss/fear event and the phobia and demonstrate

that this is a way of *re-evoking the emotional experience and memories* in the here and now. The question is: Why is it compellingly important to "remember" Barney that way now? The therapist must be aware that *some fantasies are constructed by the mind and screen other, earlier traumatic experiences.* In regard to anxiety responses to interpersonal losses, the symptoms may carry the meaning of not feeling comfortable or at least "OK" to "live" without the lost object. The degree to which these fantasies are in keeping with parents' or siblings' fantasies must be considered and articulated.

4. The aim of this work on the presenting symptoms is then to elaborate the underlying, symbolic (emotionally-relevant) "story" of the phobic/avoidant symptoms, to help the child have a way of representing them as magical (irrational) fantasy-driven reactions that started at some point—a point that has specific emotional meaning—*and has been adopted not because of a "real-world" danger but because of attachment to what the fears represent. This has ceased to be a conscious association, but the symbolic connection keeps the thoughts alive.* The process of discussing anxious thoughts and feelings repeatedly with another person in psychotherapy has the effect of *altering them to be verbally-encoded thoughts, or "mentalized";* that is, the inner reality of the child is set alongside the verbally communicated perspective of the adult (the therapist), who listens respectfully to the child's point of view and then places it alongside his/her perspective, offering the possibility of integrating the two (translating symptoms, which are symbolic representations, into words). This process of mentalizing phobic preoccupations helps to move them *out of "psychic equivalence," in which fantasies are treated as though they are real*, where they have been treated as dangerous and to be avoided.

6.5.4. Case: Eight-Year-Old Nina

The following case will serve as a specific example of the interplay of child patient and parents in symptom formation and expression in a phobic patient.

Nina, an eight-year-old girl, came to therapy for a variety of compelling anxiety symptoms. She was terrified to be anywhere away from her mother, to the extent that she cried most days when her mother left her at school. Her mother was also highly anxious about a number of things, including separation from Nina, although the mother seemed largely unaware of the extent of her own anxieties. Nina was frightened most of the time about numerous situations. Among other things, she was picky about which foods she would eat and tended to refuse all foods that were not beige or white with a barely conscious fear that she would have a stomachache if anything in her food were "unusual." Nina suffered from frequent stomachaches, although she admitted that it was often difficult to distinguish whether the problem was a "real stomach problem," like the flu, which she had had the previous winter, or whether she was "just nervous," like when her mother left her at school. Of note, Nina had a history of "severe milk allergy" with an inability to tolerate most feedings when she was several months old. This early childhood feeding problem had set a pattern of stomach worries for her as well as for mother about her.

Nina was particularly scared of Halloween and had a long-standing fear of witches ever since she had seen *The Little Mermaid* in preschool. Most Halloweens were marked by her "hiding" in her apartment, avoiding trick-or-treaters, and decorating her apartment in a complicated cross between "nice" and "scary" themes.

On the Halloween that fell two months after she began CAPP, Nina announced that she wanted to go trick-or-treating with a family friend, accompanied by her mother, in her apartment building. Much of her therapy became consumed by this plan. Nina planned her costume, which she sometimes wanted to be "a scary witch," which often frightened her as she spoke/screamed about it, or sometimes a "pretty witch," which seemed less frightening. Sometimes she thought she wanted to avoid the witch problem entirely and "just be a pilgrim." Of note, despite supporting this plan, her mother sounded anxious about Halloween and had been warning Nina not to "gorge" on candy. It was with great excitement and trepidation that she left the therapist's office the evening before Halloween.

In the next session, Nina reported that she had had a "terrible" Halloween.

THERAPIST: What happened? You've been so excited for so long.

NINA: I ate too much candy and I got a stomachache.

THERAPIST: What made you think eating candy would give you a stomachache?

NINA: Mommy said so—she said that was why I had the stomachache.

THERAPIST: Do you think you were nervous about trick-or-treating?

NINA: I don't know.

THERAPIST: How much candy did you actually have?

NINA: Two pieces.

THERAPIST: Two pieces . . .do you think that is a lot of candy?

NINA: (thoughtful) . . . I guess kids eat a lot of candy on Halloween. . . Heather did, and she was fine (laughing). So why did I have a stomachache then?

THERAPIST: What do you think about that?

NINA: I don't know.

THERAPIST: Is it possible that you were nervous being out at night for the first time on Halloween?

NINA: Maybe. And Mommy kept warning me about the candy. . . .

THERAPIST: This has been very scary for you in the past—I know you're big now, but think of last year.

NINA: I think so too (giggles). I'm going home to eat some candy!

This example demonstrates how an anxious preoccupation of the mother's has a profound anxiety-inducing effect on this separation-anxious, phobic child. The therapist realistically discusses the fantasy nature of the fear (of eating too many candies) and links it to a larger fear (of being out at night on Halloween for the first time, which to this child felt like a dangerous separation from home and her routine). The therapist does not specifically label mother's worry as unrealistic, but she implies that her reasoning may be expanded to other past reasons for avoidance and symptoms.

References

1. Deutsch, H. (1928). The genesis of agoraphobia. *International Journal of Psychoanalysis, 10*, 51–69.
2. Shapiro, T., & Jegede, R. O. (1973). School phobia: A babel of tongues. *Journal of Autism and Developmental Disorders, 3*(2), 168–186.
3. Busch, F. N., Milrod, B. L., Singer, M. B., & Aronson, A. C. (2011). *Manual of panic focused psychodynamic psychotherapy—eXtended Range*. New York, NY: Routledge.

6.6. Posttraumatic Stress Disorder With Case Vignette

6.6.1. Symptoms, Signs, and Diagnostic Considerations

Symptom onset in PTSD, by definition, occurs after exposure to a traumatic event that is extreme, meeting DSM-5 criterion A, which occurs outside of normal, expectable events. The traumatic event is defined as a severe trauma in which there is an actual or threatened death or serious physical injury or a threat to physical integrity of oneself or others (1). Being bullied persistently in childhood and/or adolescence can be traumatic enough to meet criterion A of PTSD.

Clinical similarities between panic disorder and PTSD include frequent panic attacks, a high degree of baseline anxiety, and the tendency to avoid distressing or anxiety-producing stimuli (2). In clinical situations with children and adolescents, anxiety symptoms can be difficult to untangle as "belonging" to one syndrome or another because overwhelming anxiety can become free-floating and pervasive. This may be particularly true in people who survive catastrophic trauma (2, 3). Furthermore, separation anxiety is a specific risk factor for development of PTSD in children exposed to traumatic events (4, 5) and among adults as well (6). Crucial differences between PTSD and panic disorder are both the pervasive sense of numbing that is a hallmark of PTSD, as well as the tendency to re-experience actual, psychologically vibrant elements of the traumatic experience in PTSD.

The acute anxiety states that occur in PTSD can also be experienced as arising "out of the blue," as they do in panic disorder. This type of overwhelming anxiety, in which the content of the anxiety trigger becomes disconnected from the affect, develops from the process of dissociation, a key defensive organizing feature of PTSD (7). *Dissociation can be understood in part as an unsuccessful unconscious attempt at psychological avoidance of fear-associated affects in reaction to traumatic events or as denial of the central significance of the trauma.* While patients with panic disorder can also be prone to dissociation, this tends to occur with less severity than after catastrophic or life-threatening trauma, and in panic disorder, the dissociation is generally limited to panic experiences. In both groups of patients, dissociation may be thought of as an adaptive response to overwhelming threats to personal integrity at the time the threat existed. This mode of "adaptation" ceases to be beneficial when the real threat and its associated risks recede. *For both disorders, psychodynamic interventions focus on unconscious repressed mental contents and intrapsychic conflicts that contribute to symptomatology in an effort to connect warded-off fantasies and emotions with current feelings and thoughts. In PTSD, some of these core warded off thoughts may be related to core aspects of the abuse experience (i.e., tolerating/beginning to accept that mommy in fact did beat you, for example.)*

Factors Contributing to Pretrauma Vulnerability to PTSD

Although most people (50% to 90%) encounter trauma during their lifetime (8, 9), only about 8% develop PTSD (10). Vulnerability to PTSD involves an interaction of biological diathesis, early childhood developmental experiences, and trauma type and severity. Childhood trauma, chronic adversity, and familial stressors have been found to increase risk for PTSD and for its biological markers after a traumatic event in adulthood (11, 12, 13).

Dysregulated attachment styles may increase later risk for developing anxiety disorders, including PTSD. Fraley and colleagues (14) found that survivors ($N = 45$) with secure attachment who had significant exposure to the events of September 11, 2001 described fewer PTSD and depressive symptoms on follow-up than those with insecure attachment. Attachment was assessed with the 30-item Relationship Scales Questionnaire (RSQ) (15). Twaite and Rodriguez-Srednicki (16), who studied 284 New Yorkers affected by 9/11, found that history of childhood sexual or physical abuse increased the likelihood, but secure attachment decreased the likelihood, of developing PTSD symptoms. Secure attachment potentially protected against the development of PTSD. Furthermore, separation anxiety, which necessarily involves insecure, or dysregulated attachments, predisposes to development of PTSD with trauma (6). *Thus premorbid insecure attachment and difficulty in establishing basic trust (17), due to biological predisposition and/or early life experiences, including trauma, leaves individuals vulnerable to developing PTSD.* These vulnerabilities inevitably surface in the therapeutic relationship.

6.6.2. Psychodynamic Factors and Conflicts
The Impact of Trauma on Mind and Self

Neurosecretory and psychological influences that occur during trauma experiences disrupt memory consolidation (18). Moments of terrifying clarity accompanying flashbacks alternate with disparate and often inconsistent impressions of the traumatic event, making a coherent narrative of the trauma difficult. Affective dysregulation ensues, with children's emotions emerging unpredictably and with a sense of perplexing discontinuity from regular life. This dysregulation, accompanied by the consequent traumatic disruption of the child's developing sense of agency and physical cohesion, results in a profoundly disrupted sense of self for many trauma survivors (19, 20). Boulanger (19, 20) posits that the disrupted sense of a continuous and predictable self is the central dynamism underlying PTSD symptomatology. Understanding and articulating these central elements of the traumatic experience is crucial to working psychodynamically with patients with PTSD.

Repetition, Dissociation, Guilt, and the Counterphobic Stance

A hallmark of PTSD and a central focus of the psychoanalytic understanding of trauma (21, 22), reflected in DSM criterion B of re-experiencing the trauma (1), is that of *unconscious repetition,* whether in reality, waking fantasy, or in dreams. What has been overwhelming to the survivor and has remained unintegrated into his/her sense of reality becomes seemingly inexorably repeated. Thus the child may experience an objectively dissimilar set of circumstances as a recurrence of the trauma or may unconsciously provoke an experience reminiscent of the trauma. For example, a child who witnesses a relative having a respiratory arrest and being intubated may become preoccupied with this event when he/she has an allergy attack. A girl who is sexually abused in childhood may be repeatedly drawn to and date men who treat her roughly, or force her to have sex, hence repeating the rape experience. In the psychoanalytic literature, this process has been described as *repetition compulsion* (23).

Trauma victims defend themselves against the full implications of their traumatic experiences and the often-unbearable feelings of pain, humiliation, rage, and helplessness that accompany them through various unconscious defensive maneuvers, often including the experience of dissociative states, in which the child can feel disconnected from others, reality, or his/her own emotional state. Dissociative states can alternate with intense affects, including anxiety, triggered by reminders of the horror experienced. This pattern includes the re-emergence of painful aspects of the trauma (intrusive memories, intense emotions and flashbacks) and attempts to defend against the re-emergence of the memory or its reminders through avoidance and dissociation, such as the avoidance of certain people or activities felt to be associated with the trauma, and pervasive numbing, particularly in children (24).

Sometimes children and teens with PTSD continue to experience anxiety not only as primary neurobiological discharge or as the result of defensive failure but also because it is *connected to conscious or unconscious guilt and shame* about some aspect of the traumatic experience or their role in it, for which they feel compelled to *punish themselves.* For example, a traumatized teen may have internalized the sense of dehumanization and disgust with which they were treated by a tormentor, rapist, or assailant and may consciously still experience this as a part of himself/herself for which he/she continues to deserve to be punished or humiliated. "Survivor guilt" can result from conflicts about having survived a trauma when others died or were more severely injured (25). In addition, people can identify with the aggressor (26) and can find themselves flooded with compelling fantasies/ wishes of hurting others as they themselves were hurt. This internal effort to avoid the repulsive sense of helplessness engendered by being a victim of the trauma and *to replace their sense of helplessness with the fantasy of mastery can also trigger intense guilt and self-disgust as patients become aware of their wish to damage others.*

Some victims maintain a vigorous counter-phobic stance in order to deny the extent of the impact the trauma has had. A teenage girl, for example, who was sexually abused as a child might become promiscuous in order to actively control and ragefully punish men and also to deny the knowledge that she carries with her that she was helpless and victimized. *This counter-phobic behavior may result in the patient's repeatedly putting herself in harm's way again, making her vulnerable to revictimization, a common phenomenon in patients with PTSD.*

Additional Factors Affecting Traumatic Sequelae and the Meaning of the Traumatic Experience

Specific elements of the traumatic experience can pose difficulties and can have particular meanings for the child/teen survivor that are important to consider in a psychodynamic psychotherapy. When trauma occurs as a result of interpersonal hatred and violence, survivors face a more difficult challenge than those affected by impersonal events, such as hurricanes. For example, it is the neglect of the *people* in government toward Katrina survivors that was recounted as most traumatic as individuals struggled with feeling uncared for and enraged (27). When victims become objects of vicious, dehumanizing, and humiliating behavior on the part of a victimizer, survivors plunge into a world of "psychic equivalence." That is, horrifying, disorganizing, universal fears or fantasies (such as shoot-outs and witnessing torture) have actually been witnessed and enacted in reality and contribute to an uncanny sense of living nightmare *and a lack of perceived distinction between reality and fantasy.* Rules that normally govern human behavior were suspended. These impressions do not end when the trauma ended, but rather serve to upend the victim's sense of relationships between people as well as the victim's relationship to reality.

Past experiences of helplessness and aggression may substantially affect reactions to massive trauma. Those who suffered trauma in their past or who already felt personally insecure and unsafe before the trauma are particularly vulnerable to developing PTSD. On the other hand, past experience is distinct from the actual traumatic experience that engenders PTSD, and past feelings of trust or mistrust, safety or vulnerability, can be modified substantially by the experiencing of actual trauma. Prior trauma affects the meaning of current trauma and the underlying dynamisms in traumatized individuals (28). The conscious and unconscious meanings ascribed by the child to his traumatic experiences are crucial in fully understanding personal emotional reactions to trauma.

6.6.3. Treatment: Transdiagnostic Techniques and Specific Adaptations

The essence of a psychodynamic approach to treatment of posttraumatic symptoms lies in linking the disparate symptoms themselves: those that torment the child/teen survivor and those that leave him/her numb and withdrawn to their emotional antecedents. The need for integration parallels the integrating efforts of CAPP in linking anxiety symptoms to emotional states and underlying psychological conflicts. Particular somatic sensations, for example, may actually emerge from symbolic memory encoding of elements of the trauma. An example would be the mysterious sensation of chronic nausea following a trauma in which a child had viewed a dismembered corpse. The sense of sickening repulsion may have endured through the nausea, although the symptom is no longer consciously associated with this horrifying experience and seems to take on a life on its own. This sensation, repeated over and over, is one (non-verbal, unconscious) way of keeping the original trauma in mind. The child's sense of disconnection can be identified as deriving from the trauma and can be productively referred to as an unsuccessful protective mechanism, one that developed to disguise the child's experience of anxiety and pain yet, in its pervasiveness, serves to blunt certain emotions and make ongoing anxiety and distress seem far more confusing than they need to be. Persistence of such symptoms for any length of time will have mutative, adverse effects on many aspects of normal development.

The traumatic experience acts like a lens through which to understand the child's current experience, much as the somatic panic experience in panic disorder or preoccupying anxiety in other anxiety disorders acts like a lens to identify areas of intense conflict and departures from the child's ordinary relationship to reality and way of thinking. A child who was severely bullied will enter most new social situations with the bullies' refrains echoing in his/her ears, thereby freighting the new experience with the past. CAPP's articulation helps the child/teen to understand more clearly the specific ways in which the trauma continues to affect his/her experience of the world and relationships to others.

In addition to establishing a comprehensible psychological context and narrative for what can otherwise feel like disjunctive and confusing symptoms, in psychodynamic psychotherapy the therapist explores the meaning of various fantasies central in relationship to the therapist in order to understand better the specific emotional significance of the trauma. The therapist may be viewed, for example, as a banal bureaucrat who cannot possibly understand or care about the trauma, as a tormentor, as a cowardly bystander, as a horrified witness to degradation, as an abuser, and so forth. Helping the child/teen to see these often-unconscious reactions to himself/herself and others and to appreciate a dynamic understanding of the ramifications of the trauma's impact is essential in a dynamic approach to PTSD.

Addressing Conflicts, Guilt, and Defenses (Identification With the Aggressor and Dissociation)

Addressing defenses and underlying conflicts is a key component of the CAPP approach to treatment of PTSD. Dissociation and identification with the aggressor are prominent defenses in PTSD that, when addressed in the therapy, aid the emergence in words rather than in inchoate symptomatic experiences of frightening and conflicted aspects of the trauma, facilitating better articulation and improvement in symptoms. Guilt about anger or about survival often emerges as feelings about the trauma are explored. The following case vignette is a brief clinical example of the unfolding of some of these dynamic elements within a psychodynamic treatment of a traumatized teenager.

6.6.4. Case: Sixteen-Year-Old Amber

Amber was 16½ years old when she moved to New York from Missouri to attend a computer program/early college. She had a long history of illicit substance abuse and binge alcohol abuse and had been diagnosed with attention deficit disorder (ADD) in childhood and treated with Adderall with some success. She also had a long history of chronic anxiety without panic attacks and of sleep difficulties since early childhood. Her symptoms were aggravated by the fact that her mother suffered from severe depression, bulimia, and polysubstance abuse throughout her childhood, making her home chaotic and frightening. Nonetheless, Amber had never had a panic attack until her first year in New York after she was raped.

Amber had gone to a bar with friends and was dancing with a boy she met at the bar, whom she could only vaguely remember, in part because she had consumed a significant amount of alcohol. Later, in the hospital emergency department, it was determined that the stranger had "dosed" her drink with a "rufie." Amber "woke up" in an alley behind the bar, with torn, bloody underpants at her heels, nearly naked, and she immediately recalled, through a dense fog, the boy/man raping and beating her. She was treated in an emergency department for both HIV prevention and other sexually transmitted diseases but declined to press charges because she recalled so few specifics about her assailant because of the drug. Her parents flew in from Missouri and stayed with her.

That night, she had her first panic attack, feeling as though "the walls were coming in on me" and as if she could not locate her body on the bed. Her old childhood fears of the dark re-emerged explosively, and she was frightened and panicky, feeling as though she could disappear or die if any lights were turned off. She could not be alone. Her parents stayed with her for weeks, but she could not return to school that semester because of inability to focus and severe anxiety. She stopped taking Adderall, which helped her to concentrate at school, and refused any medication whatsoever, out of an unstated terror that she might become foggy like she did the night of the rape.

When Amber presented for psychotherapy three months after the rape, she reported her story in a monotone. Although she consciously described her current problems after she told the story of the rape, she also seemed surprised that the therapist linked her panic attacks, other anxiety symptoms, and dissociative symptoms to the rape. "But how could it affect me so deeply," Amber asked, "I don't even really remember it because of the drug he put in my drink. And anyway, I don't ever want to think about it again. Ever. I'm not discussing it." She nearly left the office.

In psychotherapy, the therapist listened to Amber telling story after story about her current life, which featured ways in which Amber felt and how she was repeatedly mistreated by boyfriends. One boyfriend actually date-raped her after she broke up with him because he was threatening. The therapist was only gradually able to show Amber in real time the way that she managed to repeat many key elements of the rape experience over and over: in specific, the feeling of being "loopy" and out of control (by drinking and using drugs), a key feature of her panic experience when she had panic attacks, and the surprising, apparently out-of-the-blue vicious mistreatment by men whom she thought she could trust. It was only after her second rape by her ex-boyfriend that Amber was finally able to recognize that in fact she was *"remembering" the rape constantly, over and over, without actually permitting herself "to think" about it consciously or discuss it in words.* It was only at this point that she was able to begin to change the way she thought about and approached relationships with men and that her severe panic and PTSD experiences improved.

Therapist's Understanding of Amber's PTSD Symptomatology

This example demonstrates some of the central psychodynamic underpinnings of PTSD: an ever-present, often unspoken terror that the trauma could repeat itself at the drop of a hat, which often reinforces a reluctance to recall and discuss it, an example of dissociation and avoidance functioning defensively. While thinking about the traumatic event can sometimes be avoided consciously, the patient's preoccupation with the events expresses itself intrusively, in this case in repeated re-enactments and re-experiencing of key components of the rape. Amber felt a deep sense of humiliation and shame at having been rendered helpless, abused, and raped. She blamed herself for picking up a stranger and drinking so much. She experienced an ongoing, all-consuming struggle to regain even a relative sense of safety and self-coherence; she was plagued by often unconscious, disruptive rage at the boy/man who raped her, which spread to her feelings about men in general. As she became better able to describe her experiences with boys and men in words, she gradually became aware of her tendency to pick almost violent, irrational fights with boyfriends as a routine way of interacting with men from the very beginning of her relationships ever since her rape. This pattern tilted most romantic experiences toward men who were attracted to such behavior and introduced violent power struggles into interactions from the start.

Amber suffered from a fairly clear sense of guilt about the rape after she was able to permit herself to think about and discuss it. She was well aware that her "wild party" lifestyle (unknown to her parents, who had encouraged her to go away to school to "get away" from her friends whom they judged a "bad influence" in Missouri) was deeply irresponsible, and she blamed herself openly for what happened. "Well, I was just an idiot," she frequently said. Her guilt over her rage at her mother as well as her mother's own "wild" tendencies played a role in her unconsciously seeking punishment through the repeated re-enactments of her rape and revictimizations. These enactments were also fueled by her unconscious attempts to master the traumatic experience and to show herself and the world that she could never be so helpless and abused again. Such enactments may also have been revisitations of even earlier traumatic events, when she felt unprotected by her intoxicated mother, and her drinking may well have occurred as an identification with her mother.

This patient frequently functioned on a plane in which action reigned supreme, a not uncommon situation for some teenagers, and she literally could not permit herself to think about or understand why she engaged in many of the (posttraumatic) behaviors that she felt a sudden and unexplained urgency to do, an example of dissociation. Gradually putting her experiences into words, and then translating her seemingly inexplicable actions into an understandable frame of these experiences as being a part of her emotional response to her rape, permitted her to slowly gain distance from the rape experience itself and, specifically, helped her to become less anxious and frantic. Focusing on the transference, particularly on her chronic irritation with her therapist's emphasis on verbalizing her experiences, and working through her traumatic response to the rape also enabled her to resurrect traumatic memories from childhood, including those of her traumatic attachment to her mother, and to begin to explore the possibility of new relationships in which she could allow herself to begin to trust another person in a different way.

Length of Psychodynamic Psychotherapy for PTSD

Some of the teenagers in our clinical trial of CAPP (29) had comorbid PTSD that remitted with 24 sessions of CAPP, although none of them had primary PTSD.

Some authors (22, 30, 31) have emphasized that to fully treat complex PTSD, an open-ended, long-term psychodynamic psychotherapy or psychoanalysis is necessary. This recommendation is based on the clinical experience that for multiply or deeply traumatized individuals, a sufficiently trusting alliance often develops only very gradually, over time, because of the victim's inherent mistrust of others and that some of the most trenchant and hidden elements of the traumatic schemata are unlikely to reveal themselves within a brief treatment. Sexually traumatized individuals may find themselves excited by danger, aggravating retraumatization and making motivation for change at best mixed. Some authors (32, 33) caution that expressive and interpretive work exposing PTSD patients to the full affective force of their experience may be unproductive or even dangerous for patients with unstable relationship and work/school histories before their trauma and for those who have difficulty with self-observation (34). Regardless of the duration of the psychotherapy, clinicians need to perform ongoing evaluations of the child/teen's responses to the interventions.

Psychodynamic treatments can help patients to develop insight and improved mentalization capacities, key deficits that form a part of the nidus of the anxiety and posttraumatic syndrome.

References

1. American Psychiatric Association. (2013). *Diagnostic and statistical manual of mental disorders* (5th ed.). Washington, DC: American Psychiatric Press.
2. North, C. S., Suris, A. M., Davis, M., & Smith, R. P. (2009). Toward validation of the diagnosis of posttraumatic stress disorder. *American Journal of Psychiatry, 166,* 34–41.
3. Cougle, J. R., Feldner, M. T., Keough, M. E., Hawkins, K. A., & Fitch, K. E. (2010). Comorbid panic attacks among individuals with posttraumatic stress disorder: Associations with traumatic event exposure history, symptoms, and impairment. *Journal of Anxiety Disorders, 24,* 183–188.

4. Laor, N., Wolmer, L., Mayes, L. C., Gershon, A., Weizman, R., & Cohen, D. J. (1996). Israeli preschoolers under Scud missile attacks: A developmental perspective on risk-modifying factors. *Archives of General Psychiatry, 53*(5), 416–423.

5. Saxe, G. N., Stoddard, F., Hall, E., Chawla, N., Lopez, C., Sheridan, R., . . . Yehuda, R. (2005). Pathways to PTSD, part I: Children with burns. *American Journal of Psychiatry, 162*(7), 1299–1304.

6. Silove, D., Alonso, J., Bromet, E., Gruber, M., Sampson, N., Scott, K., . . . Kessler, R. C. (2015). Pediatric-onset and adult-onset separation anxiety disorder across countries in the World Mental Health Survey. *American Journal of Psychiatry, 172*(7), 647–656.

7. Anderson, F. S., & Gold, J. (2003). Trauma, dissociation, and conflict: The space where neuroscience, cognitive science, and psychoanalysis overlap. *Psychoanalytic Psychology, 20*, 536–541.

8. Kessler, R. C., Sonnega, A., Bromet, E., Hughes, M., & Nelson, C. B. (1995). Posttraumatic stress disorder in the National Comorbidity Survey. *Archives of General Psychiatry, 52*, 1048–1060.

9. Breslau, N., Kessler, R. C., Chilcoat, H. D., Schultz, L. R., Davis, G. C., & Andreski, P. (1998). Trauma and posttraumatic stress disorder in the community: The 1996 Detroit Area Survey of Trauma. *Archives of General Psychiatry, 55*, 626–632.

10. Alexander, P. C., & Anderson, C. (1994). An attachment approach to psychotherapy with the incest survivor. *Psychotherapy, 31*, 665–675.

11. Koenen, K. C., Moffitt, T. E., Poulton, R., Martin, J., & Caspi, A. (2007). Early childhood factors associated with the development of post-traumatic stress disorder: Results from a longitudinal birth cohort. *Psychological Medicine, 37*, 181–92.

12. Otte, C., Neylan, T. C., Pole, N., Metzler, T., Best, S., Henn-Haase, C., . . . Marmar, C. R. (2005). Association between childhood trauma and catecholamine response to psychological stress in police academy recruits. *Biological Psychiatry, 57*, 1, 27–32.

13. Resnick, H. S., Yehuda, R., Pitman, R. K., & Foy, D. W. (1995). Effect of previous trauma on acute plasma cortisol level following rape. *American Journal of Psychiatry, 152*(11), 1675–1677.

14. Fraley, R. C., Fazzari D. A, Bonanno, G. A., & Dekel, S. (2006). Attachment and psychological adaptation in high exposure survivors of the September 11th attack on the World Trade Center. *Personality and Social Psychology Bulletin, 32*, 538–551.

15. Griffin, D. W., & Bartholomew, K. (1994). The metaphysics of measurement: The case of adult attachment. In K. Bartholomew & D. Perlman (Eds.), *Advances in personal relationships: Vol. 5. Attachment processes in adulthood* (pp. 17–52). London, UK: Jessica Kingsley.

16. Twaite, J. A., & Rodriguez-Srednicki, O. (2004). Childhood sexual and physical abuse and adult vulnerability to PTSD: The mediating effects of attachment and dissociation. *Journal of Child Sexual Abuse, 13*, 17–38.

17. Fonagy, P., & Bateman, A. (2008). The development of borderline personality disorder—A mentalizing model. *Journal of Personality Disorders, 22*, 4–21.

18. LeDoux, J. (2002). *Synaptic self.* New York, NY: Penguin Books.

19. Boulanger, G. (2002). Wounded by reality: The collapse of the self in adult onset trauma. *Contemporary Psychoanalysis, 38*, 45–76.

20. Boulanger, G. (2007). *Wounded by reality: Understanding and treating adult onset trauma.* Hillsdale, NJ: Analytic Press.

21. Freud, S. (1946). *The ego and the mechanisms of defense.* New York, NY: International Universities Press.

22. Lindy, J. (1996). Psychoanalytic psychotherapy of posttraumatic stress disorder: The nature of the therapeutic relationship. In B. van der Kolk, A. McFarlane, & L. Weisaeth (Eds.), *Traumatic stress: The effects of overwhelming experience on mind, body, and society* (pp. 525–536). New York, NY: Guilford.

23. Corradi, R. B. (2009). The repetition compulsion in psychodynamic psychotherapy. *Journal of the American Academy of Psychoanalysis, 37*, 477–500.

24. Terr, L. (1992). *Too scared to cry.* New York, NY: Basic Books.

25. Krupnick, J. L., & Horowitz, M. J. (1981). Stress response syndromes: Recurrent themes. *Archives of General Psychiatry, 38*(4), 428–435.

26. Freud, A. (1946). *The ego and the mechanisms of defense.* New York, NY: International Universities Press.

27. Lee, S. (2006). *When the levees broke: A requiem in four acts* (documentary film).

28. Caruth, C. (1996). *Unclaimed experience: Trauma, narrative and history.* Baltimore, MD: Johns Hopkins University Press.

29. Milrod, B., Shapiro, T., Gross, C., Silver, G., Preter, S., Libow, A., & Leon, S. C. (2013). Does Manualized Psychodynamic Psychotherapy have an impact on youth anxiety disorders? *American Journal of Psychotherapy*, *67*(4), 359–366.

30. Weiss, D. S., & Marmar, C. R. (1993). Teaching time-limited dynamic psychotherapy for post-traumatic stress disorder and pathological grief. *Psychotherapy Research*, *30*, 587–591.

31. Kudler, H. S., Blank, A. S., & Krupnick, J. L. (2004). Psychodynamic therapy. In E. B. Foa, T. M. Keane, & M. J. Friedman (Eds.), *Effective treatments for PTSD* (pp. 176–198). New York, NY: Guilford.

32. Krystal, H. (1988). *Integration and self-healing: Affect, trauma, alexithymia*. Hillsdale, NJ: Analytic Press.

33. Gabbard, G. O. (2000). *Psychodynamic psychiatry in clinical practice* (3rd ed.). Washington, DC: American Psychiatric Press.

34. Rudden, M. G., Milrod, B., Meehan, K. B., & Falkenstrom, F. (2009). Symptom-specific reflective functioning: Incorporating psychoanalytic measures into clinical trials. *Journal of the American Psychoanalytic Association*, *57*, 1473–1478.

7

Course of Marie's Treatment

Opening, Middle, and Termination Phases

We conclude this manual with the presentation of Marie's treatment.

Marie, who we met at the beginning of the manual, is a 14-year-old ninth-grader who presented with a two-and-a-half-year history of severe anxiety, episodes of dizziness and crying, and inability to speak in situations outside of her home or school classes. She refused to leave her house alone for fear of "seeing someone" and possibly needing to interact with them, albeit with just a wave. Her greatest fears concerned seeing kids her own age, even from a distance. She said she had also become "too nervous" to speak to adult neighbors she had known for years. The idea of walking into a convenience store near her home and asking for something from "a stranger at a counter" felt unreachable. Her *Diagnostic and Statistical Manual of Mental Disorders, fourth edition* (DSM-IV) diagnoses at evaluation on the Anxiety Disorders Interview Schedule, Child and Parent Version (ADIS-C/P) (1) were: social phobia 7/8, agoraphobia 6/8, separation anxiety disorder 4/8, and posttraumatic stress disorder (PTSD) from severe bullying in middle school 4/8.

7.1. Evaluation, Opening Phase, and Identification of Central Dynamism

7.1.1. Evaluation

Marie's first session took place with her mother, and this was the only time her mother attended a session. The following history was obtained from both of them, with the mother doing much of the talking, and Marie nodding silently much of the time.

Marie was a shy, retiring girl with just a few close friends. She came from a close-knit, religious family. She concealed the severity of her crippling anxiety from her parents, saying she "just didn't feel like" going out. Secretly in despair, feeling trapped and incompetent, she contemplated suicide and resorted to cutting her wrists and legs to relieve tension, accompanied by thoughts of dying.

Marie had always been "shy" and serious in demeanor. She was teased at recess since starting kindergarten for being different, in particular regarding her ethnic background. During middle school, particularly seventh and eighth grades, the "teasing" from peers escalated to vicious bullying by most of the class. Day after day, anytime teachers left the room and between classes, Marie's peers turned on her "like a wolf-pack," taunting her, calling her "stupid," "ugly," "crazy," and screaming that she would be better off committing suicide. There was an ethnic-slur edge to these taunts that Marie could not repeat. One girl, a former elementary school chum who later became the bully ringleader, hit her, giving her a black eye. Marie never fought back. An adult neighbor witnessed the physical attack and reported it to Marie's mother. When Marie's mother asked her about it, however, Marie denied it, saying she had "fallen" on the street. She found the bullying deeply embarrassing, a marker for shame and humiliation. She did tell her mother "as an aside" that she wanted to switch schools. When this history was reviewed at the start of treatment, it emerged that her delivery was so offhand that her mother "never thought twice" about advising her against a switch. The school ended in eighth grade anyway, her mother reasoned, and it seemed unnecessary to change schools just for one more year. Marie continued to suffer, sobbing herself to sleep most nights, cutting more and more.

To her immense relief, Marie changed schools for ninth grade to a school in another area that specialized in the arts, something she loved. Before starting the new school, she had the fantasy that "everything would be fine" when she had the opportunity to leave her tormentors forever. Nonetheless, to her surprise, her anxiety grew even worse in the new school. Now, she felt even more unable to venture into public spaces, and she had intrusive thoughts of being ridiculed if she needed to speak at all. Marie felt ever more awkward and embarrassed about the growing chasm of what she thought she ought to be able to do as a 13-year-old, then a 14-year-old, such as going out by herself the way her peers did, and about her mounting fears of being outside of her home. She had nightly nightmares about bullies in her old school, something she did not reveal until later in therapy (during the middle phase).

Her mother finally learned about the severity of her social phobia and agoraphobia one afternoon when she tried to force Marie to go into a store alone to buy a textbook she needed. Marie refused and finally collapsed in sobs, admitting to her mother how terrified she was to go anywhere or speak to anyone, even the lady at the information desk at the store. At this point, her mother brought her for treatment.

7.1.2. Opening Phase

In the first session, Marie presented with her mother, who did most of the talking. Her mother was a loud and very expressive person, in radical contrast to Marie, who appeared mouse-like and mostly whispered politely when she was spoken to. The mother was clearly very concerned that Marie's symptoms—and the bullying—were so extreme and so extensive and that she did not know about it. The therapist used this session to try to discuss communication in the family and to try to help Marie to speak up, which was not easy. At the end of the session, Marie's mother unexpectedly announced that she and her husband might be getting a divorce. She announced this at the very end of the session, when no time was left for discussion.

In the next session, the therapist asked Marie about her feelings about her mother's announcement at the end of the session. Marie quietly reassured the therapist that her parents were not definitely getting a divorce and informed the therapist that she had left the session and cut herself on the thigh. The therapist pointed out that it might have been difficult for Marie to leave the office with the threat of her parents' divorce suddenly expressed with no time to respond. Marie said she was embarrassed about cutting herself, and the therapist spent time exploring in detail Marie's feelings when she cut herself. Cutting seemed to serve a soothing role for her, yet it also reinforced a feeling about herself as being "crazy" and "bad," like the bullies had labeled her.

Over the next several sessions, Marie spoke shyly about how loud and embarrassing her mother was. She clearly felt quite uncomfortable bringing this up and took back most of what she said almost as she said it. Nonetheless, the therapist linked Marie's embarrassment about mother's loudness with Marie's own shyness and wish to be different from mother, bringing elements of Marie's *social phobia into focus as a specific wish to delineate herself as being separate from her mother.* Marie agreed that this was very important to her.

Clinical Encounter

MARIE: It's fine for her, that's her personality.

THERAPIST: Right, but it sounds like you're also saying that it embarrasses you.

MARIE: I know I should try and be more accepting of her as a person, I can't help being embarrassed.

THERAPIST: How upsetting is it to you?

Over the next sessions, Marie elaborated on the extreme humiliation she felt about her mother's brashness and constant calling attention to herself in public, behaviors that made Marie want to disappear "down a drain." It emerged that one aspect of her former classmates' bullying of her had been about how "weird" her family was. These taunts had left Marie feeling torn: she secretly agreed that her mother was embarrassing, but she automatically defended her mother in her mind.

At their fourth session, Marie came in quite upset and anxious. Her mother had become enraged at her on the subway going home from the therapist's office after the last session when Marie had asked her to "please talk less loudly," something she rarely dared to do, but had ventured to say in part because of the embarrassment about her mother that she had been discussing in her therapy. That was several days previously, and Marie's mother had not spoken to her since.

Clinical Encounter

THERAPIST: Was that really the whole fight?

MARIE: Yes, it's the whole thing.

THERAPIST: Well, what do you think about your mom's reaction to what you said?

MARIE: . . . I don't know. Maybe she's a little bit overreacting.

THERAPIST: I agree. You really didn't say anything mean to her?

MARIE: I guess not. But I'm so upset now, I'm feeling even more anxious.

THERAPIST: So how unusual is this overreaction of your mom's?

Throughout the next several sessions, the therapist explored more underpinnings of Marie's reticence. It emerged that living in her home was like "walking on eggshells," with her mother almost always "fit to explode" at very small criticisms by anyone in the family. "I just have learned to shut up and keep to myself," Marie said sadly, noting again that her bullies made fun of her mother's brashness to her.

Meanwhile, Marie remained frightened to leave her home without her mother or her best friend accompanying her. Much time was spent on her fears, which revolved around recurrent thoughts of seeing her middle school bullies again, who all lived in her neighborhood, and feeling that if she saw them she would have to run away, which would only further humiliate her and make her feel stupid and inadequate.

7.1.3. Identification of Central Dynamism

At this point in the therapy, it had become clear and specifically articulated by the therapist that what underlay Marie's shyness was not only her very conscious wish to be the "opposite" of her loud, brash, and embarrassing mother but also a style that was heavily reinforced by her mother's extreme negative rage reactions to any expression of disapproval of her by Marie. Marie had been taught to hold her temper by her mother through her rage attacks, so tension ran high. Marie was barely conscious of her disapproval of her mother much of the time, which made her feel guilty. All of this contributed to her sense that she could not speak up or defend herself.

7.2. Middle Phase

The exploration of the dynamisms underlying Marie's anxiety and agoraphobia was the main focus of the middle phase.

Clinical Encounter

MARIE: It's so pathetic, it's like their opinion of me has permanently marked me. It's so unfair.

The therapist explored Marie's fantasies about what she would like to say to the bullies if she were to see them.

> MARIE: I'd be scared I couldn't say anything is the problem. That would just prove to them that they were always right to judge me like that.
>
> THERAPIST: So saying nothing, like you did all those years, sounds like it would be the worst. That terrifies you.
>
> MARIE: The worst.
>
> THERAPIST: What if you managed to speak?
>
> MARIE: I never thought of that. I guess I would want to say: "I don't care about you."
>
> THERAPIST: OK.
>
> MARIE: (covers her face) It feels too brave to me. I don't know why. (long pause) It might matter which one of them I ran into. Like William or Marissa, well I don't know—they really are nobody. I really honestly don't care what they think about anything. They're hypocrites.
>
> THERAPIST: OK—who's the absolute worst?
>
> MARIE: Oh my goodness, Amanda! Amanda used to be my friend! Then she's the one who beat me up. She was the ringleader of everyone who bullied me. No matter whatever was happening, Amanda was always in my face, putting me down relentlessly, telling me to kill myself. It's what she lived for!
>
> THERAPIST: So she's really important.
>
> MARIE: Oh my gosh. I've been having these dreams about her almost every night.

Marie then reported recurrent dreams of trying to escape Amanda, who continued to bully her. The dreams turned vicious, and Marie repeatedly found herself physically assaulting Amanda, "ripping her face off so there was blood on my nail polish!" The dreams often took place in her church. Marie hid her face and spoke in whispers as she reported these dreams in a rush, ending with, "I'm a terrible person!"

> THERAPIST: Well, I guess I'm starting to see why you may have been frightened of speaking up and defending yourself. I think you have been terrified of how understandably furious you are at these bullies, especially Amanda, who was your friend when you were small, and you're pretty frightened of how angry you get.
>
> MARIE: I know!

This session, the report of the nightmares, and *Marie's beginning acknowledgment of her murderous rage at the bullies, and so many other people, who she viewed as phonies, including religious leaders whom her mother admired, was a turning point in her therapy.* Gradually at this point, Marie expanded her life, traveling to and from her therapy sessions on her own and going out of her way to be more social with new kids. She was beginning to enjoy being more independent and to feel more comfortable having opinions that differed from her mother or her friends.

7.3. Termination Phase

Toward the end of the therapy, Marie was very anxious, yet auditioned and was accepted for the part of "white girl" in a play at her school about bullying and racism. With great trepidation, she stood up in front of her class and told the class about her experience being bullied. "If I can't let myself do this while I'm still in therapy, with you to come and talk to, when will I ever let myself do this?" she pointed out one day. The class and teacher's positive response to and support of her increased her sense of confidence.

This patient openly dreaded her therapy ending, but she did not develop a recrudescence of her anxiety symptoms. Instead, she spent time focusing on trying to incorporate her anger and disappointment with her mother and others in her community into "the way I think about my life." She articulated a few things she wanted to be able to do without anxiety, such as confronting her priest about the church's position on homosexuality, and she was pleased to report being able to begin to broach the subject with him. She lost her DSM diagnoses at treatment termination and remained well at the eight-month follow-up, free of anxiety.

7.4. Summary

Marie came to therapy riddled with anxious inhibitions arising from her traumatic history of being bullied, leading to PTSD. Bullying had occurred as an overlay to her chronically (lifelong) style of not being able to speak up for herself, not defending herself, and avoiding and disavowing her negative feelings across the board, most prominently in her relationship with her domineering, loud, and irritable mother.

In her therapy, Marie was able to articulate her mixed and angry feelings about her mother and, more importantly, about her bullies. Being able to openly acknowledge her murderous rage, as was illustrated in her recurrent dreams of physically assaulting Amanda, was a turning point in allowing her to take a more active and self-protective role in her own life. She used termination to shore up her abilities to confront people who made her angry in her life, and the treatment resulted in her losing all of her DSM diagnoses and living a much more satisfying life.

Reference

1. Silverman, W. K., & Albano, A. M. (2004). *Anxiety disorders interview schedule (ADIS-IV), child parent version*. New York, NY: Oxford University Press and Graywind Publications.

Glossary

Basic Psychodynamic Concepts

Central psychodynamic concepts are important to an understanding of the psychodynamic theory of anxiety disorders and to using child and adolescent anxiety psychodynamic psychotherapy (CAPP). These concepts are the building blocks that form underpinnings of clinical meaning of patients' symptoms, fantasies, and conflicts and inform psychodynamic interventions. There is some overlap between many of these concepts that have been altered over time and are dynamic in their use. They are not meant to be rigid categories.

Intrapsychic Factors
Unconscious Thought

Freud, the originator of our psychodynamic frame, posited that psychic content is either readily available to consciousness or exists in a more inaccessible realm initially described as "the unconscious" (1). Emotional material (fantasies, feelings, wishes) are unconsciously kept out of awareness (2), or repressed, because they are experienced as painful, frightening, or unacceptable. These intrapsychic contents are referred to as the dynamic unconscious, which implies that psychic contents that are unconscious remain so for a dynamic (i.e., emotionally meaningful) reason, because of the *emotional danger they represent* to the stability of the ego. Individuals typically experience the emergence into consciousness of these unconscious wishes, fantasies, or feelings as potentially threatening to their safety or well-being or as morally unacceptable. *Conflict between wishes or fantasies and prohibitions against them is referred to as intrapsychic conflict, a central psychodynamic principle.* The mind is in a state of well-being when the amount of intrapsychic conflict is low; this is the normal state of affairs.

Well-being can be preserved as long as new triggers for tension can be tolerated and adapted to. However, when significant conflict about specific feelings and fantasies are stirred up, or frustration of wishes by external factors is experienced, emotionally engendered symptoms can be triggered. A significant change in Freud's model was introduced when the unconscious was no longer designated as a theoretical space, and unconscious became an adjective, as in "unconscious fantasy," indicating out of awareness (3). In this newer model, fantasies were kept out of awareness because *"signal anxiety"* was aroused. Signal anxiety occurs when the ego senses danger in emergent fantasies, and *signals* the presence of danger. After this "signal," defenses are triggered actively to maintain internal equilibrium in "*compromise formations*," which lead to symptoms. Throughout this manual, intrapsychic conflicts that trigger anxiety symptoms, agoraphobia, and other panic-like events are viewed from this perspective.

For example, patients with panic attacks and severe anxiety are often entirely unaware of angry feelings toward others to whom they feel closely attached. These fantasies and the associated feelings remain largely unconscious, and any emerging awareness triggers anxiety and a host of avoidant mental responses, the purpose of which is to prevent any further awareness, enactment, or expression of the unacceptable, seemingly dangerous wishes. The expression of anger is imagined to endanger and disrupt the relationship, which is felt to be essential for security and coherence (4, 5). A central component of psychodynamic treatment, and of CAPP, is helping children and adolescents to gain access to aspects of their unconscious mental lives that trigger maladaptive patterns and symptoms. Symptoms diminish as wishes, fantasies, and conflicts become conscious, are better understood, and are able to be expressed in verbal form. Unconscious fantasies (2), that often relate to past experiences from earlier development and contain wishes that are a source of conflict and discomfort, can play an important role in panic and anxiety symptoms.

Defense Mechanisms

Unacceptable or frightening unconscious fantasies and feelings are screened from consciousness, following small traces of signal anxiety by psychological processes called defense mechanisms (6) that operate outside of consciousness.

An example of a defense mechanism is *denial,* a process in which the individual disavows the perception of a compelling, uncomfortable feeling or fantasy. An example of the use of denial is anxiety patients' lack of awareness of angry feelings and fantasies. For example, children and adolescents with anxiety disorders may disavow angry feelings at someone even though they have just expressed them, or they may not acknowledge anger at a friend even though anger might be appropriate in the situation in which they find themselves. Negation by contrast is a linguistic tool by which one may consciously deny a conscious perception.

In addition to denial, other defense mechanisms found prominently among patients with anxiety disorders in studies and clinical observations include *reaction formation* and *undoing*; both are similarly utilized in the child's unconscious management of overwhelming ambivalence and separation fears. *Reaction formation* involves the apparent conversion of unacceptable feelings into their opposite, such as anger into excessive concern.

Patients may demonstrate an excessive effort to help others with whom they would be expected to be angry.

In the process of *undoing*, an individual symbolically makes amends for the internal experience or outward expression of a conflicted wish or fantasy, usually an angry one. Shakespeare's line, "The lady doth protest too much, methinks" (*Hamlet,* Act 3, Scene 2) represents an apt response to reaction formation. One example of this process involves patients "taking back" angry comments they have made about another person, thereby reassuring themselves that the terror they experience that such a comment might endanger the relationship no longer exists. *Somatization* is a ubiquitous defense in panic and anxiety disorders, particularly among children and adolescents, as unacceptable feelings and fantasies are avoided unconsciously and are instead experienced as disturbing bodily sensations such as stomachaches rather than as emotional events. Sometimes physical symptoms can symbolize unconscious fantasies.

In CAPP, the therapist seeks to identify the presence and meanings of defenses as early in the encounter as possible and shares these with the patient, with the goal of exploring underlying conflicted fantasies that trigger symptoms and resolving the conflicts in a more adaptive way (7).

Compromise Formation

A compromise formation (1) is a ubiquitous, unconscious process of mental life that symbolically represents a compromise between an unacceptable wish and the defense against that wish. Symptoms, dreams, fantasies, and aspects of personality can be productively understood as compromise formations. Panic attacks and other anxiety symptoms often represent a compromise between unacceptable or frightening aggressive fantasies, conflicted dependency wishes, and self-punishment for these fantasies. The aggressive wishes emerge in patients' coercive efforts to control others whom the patient feels are necessary for his/her safety but toward whom he/she has ambivalent feelings. Unacknowledged and unacceptable dependency wishes can be expressed in this way, as the patient's wishes for attention and comfort are communicated indirectly through help-seeking for fantasized physical problems or even anxiety symptoms *per se*. The patient's terror and disability function in part as self-punishment for these forbidden wishes. Brenner's (8) daring revision of psychodynamic theory endorses compromise formation as the spare minimal essential of the psychoanalytic model.

Representation of Self and Others

In the course of development, individuals form internalized (inner mental) representations of themselves and of others with whom they have significant relationships. This theoretical beginning involves separation–individuation (9) as well as identification and the early definition of the self (10). Definition of the self is more coherent if it arises in situations within secure, primary attachment relationships, which most commonly occurs in mother-child dyads featuring "good-enough mothering" (11), as well as appropriate escape from narcissism and the ability to acknowledge and love others without regressive primitive responses to perceived slights and fantasied betrayal. The nature and development of these representations play an important role in the emergence of symptoms. Internalized models of formative central relationships continue to shape the way people see relationships, what they anticipate, and how they behave toward others. Clinical and research evidence suggests that patients who are vulnerable to severe anxiety and panic attacks have particular patterns of internalized representations, including expectations of control, overprotection, and rejection (12, 13, 14). Clinically, they frequently describe caregivers who were frightening, temperamental, and judgmental. Based on these templates, patients often anticipate that their relationships will be easily disrupted and that a range of feelings and experiences, particularly surrounding separation and anger, are unsafe because they could too easily result in the rupture of the relationship.

Mentalization

Mentalization refers to the capacity to conceive of behavior and emotion in terms of mental states in oneself and others (15). Its developmental precursor is Theory of Mind. This emergent capacity to stand apart from experience and also to view one's self is akin to Sterba's (16) psychoanalytically derived notion of the Observing Ego. For patients with anxiety disorders, the poor acknowledgment about internal, emotional contributors to anxiety symptoms can be viewed as a focal impairment in mentalization. Patients often report "not knowing" in an unconscious effort to avoid frightening feelings and fantasies. Thus panic and anxiety symptoms can feel as if they arise "out of the blue." CAPP treatment in part helps patients to improve their capacity to mentalize and consider their anxiety symptoms reflectively. Such improved capacity fosters greater understanding about the relationship between anxiety, underlying emotional life, and conflicts and how they are triggered by the stressors. Reflective functioning (15) refers to an operationalized, measurable dimension of the capacity for mentalization. A measure of symptom-specific reflective functioning (SSRF) has been developed by Rudden et al. (17, 18) for the purpose of assessing this capacity, specifically about psychic symptoms. Patients with panic disorder experienced improvements in SSRF after panic-focused psychodynamic psychotherapy (PFPP) (19, 20).

Clinical Manifestations

Symptoms

From a psychodynamic perspective, symptoms are compromise formations derived in part from the threatened emergence into consciousness of frightening or unacceptable unconscious wishes, feelings, or fantasies (3).

Symptoms emerge as compromise formations, and anxiety symptoms per se contain the symbolic representation of both the expression of a forbidden wish and the defense against that wish. Thus symptoms carry unconscious, highly important symbolic meanings and symbolize central conflicted fantasies, a defense against these fantasies in somatic disguise, and they also inherently contain the punishment for unacceptable wishes (see unconscious fantasy; compromise formation). Physical symptoms can be associated with unconscious identifications with significant others. In patients who develop specific panic or acute anxiety symptoms after the death of a close attachment figure, these symptoms can come to symbolically represent the loss. As with dreams, symptoms can be understood as a developmentally earlier (preverbal and symbolic) form of mental functioning described by Freud (21) as visual and connected with immediate satisfaction of drives and wishes, marked by an absence of logic, linearity of time, and causality.

Additionally, symptoms can encapsulate contributions from specific self and object representations. Perceptions of the self as incompetent and others as rejecting and critical can heighten conflicts surrounding independence, and anxiety symptoms can include a view of the self as helpless.

Resistance

Resistance refers to the patient's unconscious efforts to oppose the therapeutic work and effects of the treatment in order to avoid the emergence of threatening unconscious fantasies or uncomfortable feelings directed toward the therapist (22). This phenomenon may take several forms, including more overt behaviors such as forgetting or coming late to appointments or expressly refusing to discuss a topic.

Resistance may emerge in more subtle forms, such as changing the subject from an uncomfortable topic or becoming silent. Efforts to rationally instruct or exhort patients to follow up on a given topic often fail because these exhortations do not address underlying reasons for resistance.

In psychodynamic treatments, resistance is seen as a valuable therapeutic marker to be understood. It is an indicator that the treatment is approaching conflicted unconscious fantasies. The therapist can address the problem by suggesting that the patient is avoiding something that appears to be embarrassing or uncomfortable. Thus resistance presents opportunities to address the emergence of conflicts in the relationship with the therapist (see Transference). Freud originally wrote of "transference resistance"—signifying that the therapeutic relationship had become a new preoccupation that enacted earlier patterns of attachment, which sought childish aims of dependence and love rather than uncovering hidden meanings that present in symptoms. Thus the regression served old unmet needs and was at the same time interfering with the job at hand of understanding.

Regression

Regression refers to a shift in thinking, adaptation, and emotional and mood states and is often patterned on behavior representing earlier developmental attachments and mechanisms (23). Regression can extend to thought processes (including a shift to primitive logic), representations of oneself and others, and fantasies.

Intrapsychic conflicts can trigger regression, which can occur generally, across many areas of functioning, or in more isolated ways. Stressors that activate underlying emotional fault lines, such as moves toward independence or interpersonal loss, can contribute to regression. Panic and other anxiety disorders frequently involve a shift to a regressed state in the expression of needy, helpless behavior. Somatization may be viewed as an anachronistic substitute for thought.

Transference

Patterns of perceptions of significant primary attachment relationships that develop in early life re-emerge in current relationships, including that with the therapist. Freud thought that the Oedipal constellation was the nuclear conflict within the earliest perceived triadic family that can be represented as a formula to describe the loving/hating, passive/active, competition for the love of the first psychological caretakers during development. This psychological phenomenon, known as transference (1, 8, 24), is a cornerstone of psychodynamic theory and practice. Awareness of and focus on the transference can be helpful to therapists and patients in articulating anachronistic organizing fantasies that surround the current therapeutic relationship, regardless of the type of treatment or the theoretical orientation of the therapist. From a psychodynamic perspective, the transference situation has far-reaching effects and necessarily influences therapeutic outcome. The transference provides both directness and immediacy in illustrating and helping to understand emotional conflicts as they come to life in the relationship. It also provides necessary conditions for the exploration of unacceptable unconscious wishes, fantasies, and feelings. Transference phenomena include both affectionate and angry feelings and fantasies, which may be experienced safely by the patient or alternatively may be a source of conflict. Affectionate feelings toward the therapist, either deriving from developmental expectations or realistically related to the therapist's role in helping the patient, can contribute to the therapeutic alliance or interfere with further uncovering of meaning (25, 26).

The therapeutic alliance constitutes the non-controversial aspects of the therapeutic relationship. Subsumed under the alliance are the sense that the patient and therapist are working collaboratively and that the therapist is empathic and the patient feels understood. In psychodynamic psychotherapy, disruptions of the therapeutic alliance are viewed as important indicators of resistance and are opportunities to address transference fantasies (27).

As transference develops in the course of CAPP, patients often experience conflicts with the therapist that are central to their anxiety.

For instance, angry feelings can develop toward the therapist in the setting of separations or termination, along with fears about losing or disrupting the relationship with the therapist. These patients are often uncomfortable getting angry, including at the therapist, and this avoidance of negative affect is likely to color the transference. Separations and termination of the treatment provide important opportunities for patients to better articulate, understand, and manage their conflicts about anger and growing autonomy in the setting of the transference.

Countertransference

Therapists develop reactions to patients based on their own internalized representations of themselves and others. This phenomenon is referred to as countertransference (28). Although countertransference can interfere with treatment, the therapist's awareness of the feelings the patient inspires in him/her can be an important clinical tool because these feelings may provide clues about the patient's behavior and state of mind. The therapist needs to remain aware of his reactions toward the patient that may be expressed directly or indirectly, such as feeling frustrated or angry, which if not acknowledged may disrupt the therapy. For example, a therapist may be drawn into a patient's sense of emergency, a common occurrence in patients with anxiety disorders, or may experience guilt about termination in connection with a patient's difficulty with separation. Sandler (29) increased our understanding of countertransference by alerting therapists to "role-responsiveness," or the tendency of the therapist to collude with the patient's transference in becoming like the patient's fantasied object within the therapeutic relationship. Such distortions become *enactments* if not recognized and confronted and do not get understood for what they represent.

References

1. Freud, S. (1955). *Studies in hysteria* (Standard ed. 2). London, UK: Hogarth Press (Originally published in 1893/1895).
2. Shapiro, T. (1992). The concept of unconscious fantasy. *Journal of Clinical Psychoanalysis, 1*, 517–524.
3. Freud, S. (1950). *Inhibitions symptoms and anxiety* (Standard ed. 20). London, UK: Hogarth Press (Originally published in 1926).
4. Busch, F. N., Cooper, A. M., Klerman, G. L., Penzer, R. J., Shapiro, T., & Shear, K. M. (1991). Neurophysiological, cognitive-behavioral, and psychoanalytic approaches to panic disorder: Toward an integration. *Psychoanalytic Inquiry, 11*(3), 316–332.
5. Shear, M. K., Cooper, A. M., Klerman, G. L., & Busch, F. N. (1993). A psychodynamic model of panic disorder. *American Journal of Psychiatry, 150*(6), 859–866.
6. Freud, S. (1911). *Formulations on the two principles of mental functioning* (Standard ed. 12, pp. 213–226). London, UK: Hogarth Press.
7. Perry, J. C., & Bond, M. (2017). Addressing defenses in psychotherapy to improve adaptation. *Psychoanalytic Inquiry, 37*, 153–166.
8. Brenner, C. (2006). *Psychoanalysis or mind and meaning.* New York, NY: Psychoanalytic Quarterly.
9. Mahler, M., & McDevitt, J. B. (1982). Thoughts on the emergence of the sense of self, with particular emphasis on the body self. *Journal of the American Psychoanalytic Association, 30*, 827–848.
10. Kohut, H., & Wolfe, E. S. (1978). The disorders of self and their treatment: An outline. *International Journal of Psychoanalysis, 59*, 413–425.
11. Winnicott, D. W. (1962). The theory of the parent-infant relationship: Further remarks. *International Journal of Psychoanalysis, 43*, 238–239.
12. Arrindell, W. A., Emmelkamp, P. M, Monsma, A., & Brilman, E. (1983). The role of perceived parental rearing practices in the aetiology of phobic disorders: A controlled study. *British Journal of Psychiatry, 143*, 183–187.
13. Silove, D. (1986). Perceived parental characteristics and reports of early parental deprivation in agoraphobic patients. *Australia and New Zealand Journal of Psychiatry, 20*(3), 365–369.

14. Parker, G. (1979). Reported parental characteristics of agoraphobics and social phobics. *British Journal of Psychiatry, 135,* 555–560.

15. Fonagy, P., Target, M., Steele H., & Steele, M. (1998). *The reflective functioning scale manual* (Version 5).

16. Sterba, R. (1934). The fate of the ego in analytic therapy. *International Journal of Psychoanalysis, 15,* 117–126.

17. Rudden, M. G., Milrod, B., Target, M., Ackerman, S., & Graf, E. (2006). Reflective functioning in panic disorder patients: A pilot study. *Journal of the American Psychoanalytic Association, 54*(4), 1339–1343.

18. Rudden, M. (2017). Reflective functioning and symptom specific reflective functioning: Moderators and mediators. *Psychoanalytic Inquiry, 37,* 129–139.

19. Milrod, B., Busch, F., Cooper, A., & Shapiro, T. (1997). *Manual of panic-focused psychodynamic psychotherapy.* Washington, DC: American Psychiatric Association Press.

20. Busch, F. N., Milrod, B. L., Singer, M. B., & Aronson, A. C. (2011). *Manual of panic focused psychodynamic psychotherapy—eXtended range.* New York, NY: Routledge.

21. Freud, S. (1953). *The interpretation of dreams* (Standard ed. 4). London, UK: Hogarth Press (Originally published in 1953).

22. Stone, L. (1975). Some problems and potentialities of present-day psychoanalysis. *Psychoanalytic Quarterly, 44,* 331–370.

23. Arlow, J. (1963). Conflict, regression and symptom formation. *International Journal of Psychoanalysis, 44,* 12–22.

24. Freud, S. (1905). *Fragment of an analysis of a case of hysteria* (Standard ed. 7, pp. 1–22). London, UK: Hogarth Press.

25. Crits-Christoph, P., Gibbons, M. C., & Mukherjee, D. (2013). Psychotherapy process-outcome research. In M. J. Lambert (Ed.), *Bergin and Garfield's handbook of psychotherapy and behavior change* (6th ed., pp. 298–340). Hoboken, NJ: Wiley and Sons.

26. Zetzel, E. R. (1956). Current concepts of transference. *International Journal of Psychoanalysis, 37,* 369–375.

27. Barber, J. P., Connolly, M. B., Crits-Christoph, P., Gladis, L., & Siqueland, L. (2000). Alliance predicts patients' outcome beyond in-treatment change in symptoms. Journal of Consulting and Clinical Psychology, 68(6), 1027–1032.

28. Gabbard, G. O. (1995). Countertransference: The emerging common ground. *International Journal of Psychoanalysis, 76,* 475–485.

29. Sandler, J. (1976). Countertransference and role responsiveness. *International Review of Psychoanalysis, 3,* 43–47.

Index